Study Guide

For

Sizer and Whitney's

Nutrition
Concepts and Controversies
Ninth Edition

Jana Kicklighter
Georgia State University

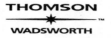
THOMSON

WADSWORTH

Australia • Canada • Mexico • Singapore • Spain • United Kingdom • United States

0-534-57800-4

**For more information about our products,
contact us at:
Thomson Learning Academic Resource Center
1-800-423-0563**

**For permission to use material from this text,
contact us by:
Phone: 1-800-730-2214
Fax: 1-800-730-2215
Web: www.thomsonrights.com**

Asia
Thomson Learning
5 Shenton Way #01-01
UIC Building
Singapore 068808

Australia
Nelson Thomson Learning
102 Dodds Street
South Street
South Melbourne, Victoria 3205
Australia

Canada
Nelson Thomson Learning
1120 Birchmount Road
Toronto, Ontario M1K 5G4
Canada

Europe/Middle East/South Africa
Thomson Learning
High Holborn House
50-51 Bedford Row
London WC1R 4LR
United Kingdom

Latin America
Thomson Learning
Seneca, 53
Colonia Polanco
11560 Mexico D.F.
Mexico

Spain
Paraninfo Thomson Learning
Calle/Magallanes, 25
28015 Madrid, Spain

CONTENTS

Chapter 5: THE LIPIDS: FATS, OILS, PHOSPHOLIPIDS, AND STEROLS

Chapter 6: THE PROTEINS AND AMINO ACIDS

Chapter 7: THE VITAMINS

Chapter 8: WATER AND MINERALS

Chapter 9: ENERGY BALANCE AND HEALTHY BODY WEIGHT

Chapter 10: NUTRIENTS, PHYSICAL ACTIVITY, AND THE BODY'S RESPONSES

Chapter 11: DIET AND HEALTH

Chapter 12: LIFE CYCLE NUTRITION: MOTHER AND INFANT

Chapter 13: CHILD, TEEN, AND OLDER ADULT

Chapter 14: FOOD SAFETY AND FOOD TECHNOLOGY

Chapter 15: HUNGER AND THE GLOBAL ENVIRONMENT

PREFACE

This *Study Guide* has been designed to accompany the ninth edition of ***Nutrition: Concepts and Controversies*** and its chapter divisions parallel those in the text. The primary goal of the *Study Guide* is to facilitate your study of the material presented in the text and enhance your learning. Pages in the *Study Guide* have been perforated and three-hole punched to enable you to insert, delete, or rearrange pages to best suit your needs or to correspond with the sequence used by your instructor.

Each chapter consists of seven sections: *chapter objectives, key concepts, a fill-in-the-blank chapter summary, chapter glossary of key terms, exercises which include chapter study questions, short answer questions, problem-solving/application questions and controversy questions, sample test items, and an answer key.* In addition, some chapters have study aids that complement material presented in the text.

To obtain the maximum benefit from this *Study Guide* you should: (1) read the chapter in the text; (2) study your class notes, and (3) complete the corresponding chapter in the *Study Guide*, including the following sections:

    Chapter Objectives and Key Concepts. Read the objectives and key concepts at the beginning of each chapter to help you focus your attention on the most essential material and concepts presented in the chapter.

    Summing Up. This section provides a brief summary of the chapter using a fill-in-the-blank format. To help you summarize and review the main points in the chapter, read the summary and fill in the blanks.

    Chapter Glossary. This section includes key terms and their definitions presented in the margins of the text. Match the definitions and terms to enhance your understanding of the material and prepare for many of the test items.

    Exercises. Chapter study questions, short answer questions, problem-solving/application questions and controversy questions are included in this section. Chapter study questions and controversy questions allow you to review key concepts and help you prepare for essay questions on examinations, while short answer and problem-solving/application questions help you to review and apply key concepts and principles presented.

    Study Aids. Many chapters include study aids to help you remember, understand and practice key information presented in the text. Some study aids refer to tables and figures in your textbook.

    Sample Test Items. Comprehension level and application level multiple choice, matching, and true/false items are included to help you test your recall and understanding of the basic content presented in the text. Many of the questions are likely to be similar to those included on examinations. However, rather than simply learning the answers to the sample test questions, you should use the questions in this section as the basis for learning and studying important concepts and principles presented in the chapter.

Answers. Answers are provided for all sections of the *Study Guide*. When checking fill-in-the-blank answers, be aware that more than one word may satisfactorily complete a sentence. If your answer differs from the one provided, determine if you have used an acceptable synonym or whether you missed the basic concept. When checking chapter study questions and controversy questions, keep in mind that only key points have been included in the answer. Good answers to discussion questions require not only a recall of the key points but also descriptions of interrelationships and explanations of why and how. A well-written answer to discussion questions requires synthesis of knowledge gained from previous lessons, related courses, and personal experience. After completing the sections of the chapter, check your answers and use your results to reinforce and strengthen the learning process by going back and restudying areas that you were unsure of or missed.

We hope you find this *Study Guide* to be useful. Please let us hear from you if you have suggestions for ways to improve the *Study Guide*.

Jana Kicklighter, Ph.D., R.D.
Department of Nutrition
Georgia State University
Atlanta, Georgia 30303

CHAPTER 1

Food Choices and Human Health

CHAPTER OBJECTIVES

After completing this chapter, you should be able to:

1. Differentiate between those diseases that are strongly influenced by diet and those that are not responsive to nutrition.

2. Identify the benefits of physical activity.

3. List the six classes of nutrients including which are organic and which are energy-yielding.

4. Describe the Dietary Guidelines for Americans.

5. Describe the process by which scientists uncover nutrition facts.

6. Describe the cultural and social meanings attached to food.

7. Identify and explain the five characteristics of a nutritious diet.

8. Begin planning a healthy diet by using the concept of nutrient density.

9. Distinguish valid nutrition information from misinformation. (Controversy 1)

KEY CONCEPTS

✓ The nutrients in food support growth, maintenance, and repair of the body. Deficiencies, excesses and imbalances of nutrients bring on the diseases of malnutrition.

✓ Nutrition profoundly affects health.

✓ Choice of diet influences long-term health, within the range set by genetic inheritance. Nutrition has no influence on some diseases but is closely linked to others.

✓ Personal life choices, such as use of tobacco or alcohol or staying physically active, also affect health for the better or worse.

✓ Food supplies energy and nutrients. The most vital nutrient is water. The energy-yielding nutrients are carbohydrates, fats (lipids), and protein. The helper nutrients are vitamins and minerals. Food energy is measured in calories; food and nutrient quantities are often measured in grams.

✓ In addition to nutrients, food conveys emotional satisfaction and hormonal stimuli that contribute to health. Foods also contain phytochemicals that give them their tastes, aromas, colors, and other characteristics. Some phytochemicals are believed to play roles in disease prevention.

✓ Foods come in a bewildering variety in the marketplace, but the foods that form the basis of a nutritious diet are staple foods such as ordinary milk and milk products; meats, fish, and poultry; vegetables and dried peas and beans; fruits; and grains.

✓ A well-planned diet is adequate in nutrients, is balanced with regard to food types, offers food energy that matches energy expended in activity, is moderate in unwanted constituents, and offers a variety of nutritious foods.

✓ Cultural traditions and social values revolve around food. Some values are expressed through foodways. Many factors other than nutrition drive food choices.

✓ The Dietary Guidelines for Americans, Nutrition Recommendations for Canadians, and other recommendations address the problems of overnutrition and undernutrition. To implement them requires exercising regularly; following the Food Guide Pyramid; amplifying servings of low-fat grains, fruits, and vegetables; limiting intakes of fats, sugar, and salt; and moderating alcohol intake.

✓ The U.S. Department of Health and Human Services sets nutrition objectives for the nation each decade.

✓ Scientists uncover nutrition facts by experimenting. Single studies must be replicated before their findings can be considered valid. New nutrition news is not always to be believed; established nutrition news has stood up to the test of time.

SUMMING UP

Nutrition is the study of how (1)_____ nourishes the body. The

human body uses (2)_____ to move and work and it comes indirectly

from the sun by way of plants. The body also requires (3)_____ kinds of

nutrients. Four of these six are (4)_____, or carbon containing. Foremost

among the six classes of nutrients in foods is (5)_____. Three of the nutrients

are energy-yielding, including carbohydrates, (6)_____, and protein.

The fifth and sixth classes of nutrients are the vitamins and (7)_____, which

act as regulators.

Some of the nutrients are (8)_____ nutrients, meaning that the body

cannot make them for itself. Special formulas are not appropriate substitutes for food because

food offers more than just the six basic (9)_____. For example, elemental

diets can support life but not optimal (10)_____ and health, and they can

often lead to medical complications. In addition, food helps maintain the intestine and conveys

messages of comfort to the (11)_____. Many compounds other than the six

classes of nutrients are also present in foods and are referred to as (12)_____.

Scientists discover nutrition facts by conducting (13)_____. Single

studies must be (14)_____ before findings can be confirmed.

Among the many factors influencing food-related choices is the (15)_____

to which a person is accustomed. People from every country enjoy special (16)_____

that represent their own heritage. Among factors people cite to explain daily food choices are

advertising, personal preference, habit, ethnic heritage, (17)_____ pressure,

availability, convenience, economy, positive associations, emotional comfort, values or beliefs,

region of the country, weight and (18)_____ value. A key to wise diet planning

is to make sure that the foods you eat daily, your (19)_____ foods, are

especially nutritious.

The U.S. Department of Health and Human Services sets ten year health objectives for the nation in its document (20) _____. Nutrition (21)_____makes it possible to assess the nutrient status and dietary intakes of the U.S. population.

An easy way to obtain a nutritious diet is to consume a (22)_____ of selections from different food groups each day. The extent to which foods support good health depends on the (23)_____, nutrients and nonnutrients they contain. A nutritious diet has five characteristics, including (24)_____, balance, calorie control, (25)_____, and variety.

CHAPTER GLOSSARY

Matching Exercise 1:

_____ 1. nutrition	a.	components of food that are indispensable to the body's functioning; they provide energy, serve as building material, help maintain or repair body parts, and support growth
_____ 2. essential nutrients		
_____ 3. food	b.	carbon containing
	c.	the study of the nutrients in foods and in the body
_____ 4. nonnutrients		
	d.	the foods (including beverages) a person eats and drinks
_____ 5. organic		
	e.	nonnutrient compounds in plant-derived foods having biological activity in the body
_____ 6. foodways		
	f.	the sum of a culture's habits, customs, beliefs, and preferences concerning food
_____ 7. energy-yielding nutrients	g.	foods associated with particular cultural subgroups within a population
_____ 8 . nutrients		
	h.	the capacity to do work
_____ 9. energy	i.	the nutrients the body cannot make for itself (or cannot make fast enough) from other raw materials
_____ 10. legumes		
	j.	the nutrients the body can use for energy
_____ 11. phytochemicals	k.	pills, liquids, or powders that contain purified nutrients or other ingredients
_____ 12. supplements	l.	medically, any substance that the body can take in and assimilate that will enable it to stay alive and to grow
_____ 13. ethnic foods		
	m.	beans, peas and lentils valued as inexpensive sources of protein, vitamins, minerals and fiber that contribute little or no fat to the diet
_____ 14. diet		
_____ 15. genome	n.	compounds other than the six nutrients that are present in foods and that have biological activity in the body
	o.	the complete set of chromosomes that comprises the entirety of an organism's genetic information

Matching Exercise 2:

_____ 1. malnutrition

_____ 2. cuisine

_____ 3. chronic diseases

_____ 4. balance

_____ 5. elemental diets

_____ 6. vegetarians

_____ 7. variety

_____ 8. calorie control

_____ 9. calories

_____ 10. grams

_____ 11. nutrient density

_____ 12. moderation

_____ 13. omnivores

_____ 14. adequacy

a. units of weight

b. diets composed of purified ingredients of known chemical composition

c. style of cooking

d. people who eat foods of both plant and animal origin, including animal flesh

e. the dietary characteristic of providing a wide selection of foods--the opposite of monotony

f. a measure of nutrients provided per calorie of food

g. any condition caused by excess or deficient food energy or nutrient intake or by an imbalance of nutrients

h. the dietary characteristic of providing all of the essential nutrients, fiber, and energy in amounts sufficient to maintain health and body weight

i. people who exclude from their diets animal flesh and possibly other animal products such as milk, cheese, and eggs

j. control of energy intake, a feature of a sound diet plan

k. the dietary characteristic of providing constituents within set limits, not to excess

l. long-duration degenerative diseases characterized by deterioration of the body organs

m. units of energy

n. the dietary characteristic of providing foods of a number of types in proportion to each other, such that foods rich in some nutrients do not crowd out of the diet foods that are rich in other nutrients

EXERCISES

Answer these chapter study questions:

1. What is meant by the statement that protein does double duty?

2. What is meant by the term essential nutrients?

3. What does food provide in addition to nutrients?

4. Why do nutrition scientists agree that people should not eat the same foods day after day?

5. Why does the variety of foods available today make it more difficult, rather than easier, to plan nutritious diets?

Complete these short answer questions:

1. The four organic nutrients include:

    a.
    b.
    c.
    d.

2. The six kinds of nutrients include:

    a.
    b.
    c.
    d.
    e.
    f.

3. The energy-yielding nutrients are:

    a.
    b.
    c.

4. Factors people cite to explain food choices include:

    a.   h.
    b.   i.
    c.   j.
    d.   k.
    e.   l.
    f.   m.
    g.   n.

5. Five characteristics of a nutritious diet include:

    a.
    b.
    c.
    d.
    e.

Solve these problems:

There are many factors which people cite to explain their food choices. For questions 1-7, match the descriptive statements on the left with the reasons for the food choices, listed on the right. The same letter is used only once.

_____ 1.   I always drink coffee at morning break.

_____ 2.   I usually microwave a frozen dinner after getting home from my night class.

_____ 3.   All my friends are going out for dessert after the play.

_____ 4.   I use dried beans as a substitute for meat because meat costs too much.

_____ 5.   I eat a lot of pasta because I like the taste.

_____ 6.   I usually choose fresh fruit for my dessert.

_____ 7.   I have to eat high fat foods because I eat in the employee cafeteria every day for lunch.

a. personal preference

b. habit

c. social pressure

d. availability

e. convenience

f. economy

g. nutritional value

Solve these controversy questions:

1.   What type of screening is required before research findings are published in scientific journals?

2.   What criterion would denote that a physician is well-qualified to speak on nutrition?

3. What is a diploma mill?

4. What are the qualifications of a dietetic technician?

5. Which type of dietetic subspecialties would you expect to see in a hospital setting?

STUDY AID

Use the following table in your textbook as a study aid: Table 1-2 on page 5.

SAMPLE TEST ITEMS

Comprehension Level Items:

1. A scientist's responsibilities include all of the following *except:*

    a.   obtaining facts by systematically asking questions
    b.   conducting experiments to test for possible answers
    c.   submitting their findings to the news media
    d.   publishing the results of their work in scientific journals

2. Which of the following nutrients is ***not*** organic?

   a. minerals
   b. vitamins
   c. protein
   d. carbohydrates
   e. fat

3. Foremost among the six classes of nutrients in foods is:

   a. fats
   b. carbohydrates
   c. vitamins
   d. water

4. Which of the following is ***not*** an energy-yielding nutrient?

   a. carbohydrates
   b. vitamins
   c. fats
   d. protein

5. All vitamins and minerals:

   a. provide energy to the body
   b. serve as parts of body structures
   c. serve as regulators
   d. are organic

6. Characteristics of essential nutrients include:

   a. the body can make them for itself
   b. they are found in all six classes of nutrients
   c. they must be received from foods
   d. a and b
   e. b and c

7. Which of the following is characteristic of elemental diets?

   a. they are sufficient to enable people to thrive
   b. they support optimal growth and health
   c. they provide everything that foods provide
   d. they are life-saving for people in the hospital who cannot eat ordinary food

8. Within the range set by your genetic inheritance, the likelihood that you will develop chronic diseases is strongly influenced by your food choices.

   a. true
   b. false

9. Which of the following is the least nutrition-responsive disease?

    a. osteoporosis
    b. hypertension
    c. low birthweight
    d. sickle-cell anemia

10. Which of the following research designs is the most powerful in pinpointing the mechanisms by which nutrition acts because it shows the effects of treatments?

    a. case studies
    b. laboratory studies
    c. epidemiological studies
    d. correlation studies

11. Which of the following is **not** a government agency responsible for monitoring the nation's nutrition?

    a. U.S. Department of Health and Human Services
    b. U.S. Department of Agriculture
    c. Food and Drug Administration
    d. Centers for Disease Control and Prevention

12. The variety of foods available today may make it more difficult, rather than easier, to plan nutritious diets.

    a. true
    b. false

13. A key to wise diet planning is to make sure your _____ foods are especially nutritious.

    a. processed
    b. fast
    c. enriched
    d. staple

14. Foods composed of parts of whole foods, such as butter, sugar, or corn oil, are called _____ foods.

    a. enriched
    b. partitioned
    c. processed
    d. staple

15. The description of a diet that provides no unwanted constituents in excess is called:

    a. variety
    b. calorie control
    c. moderation
    d. balance

16. The key to evaluating an individual food is to:

    a. judge it as either good or bad
    b. identify how it can reduce your chance of developing an illness
    c. judge its appropriate role in the context of all other food choices
    d. listen to what other people say about it

17. Foods that are rich in nutrients relative to their energy contents are called foods with high
    _____.

    a. nutrient density
    b. calorie control
    c. nutrient balance
    d. dietary moderation

18. The foods that present the most nutrients per calorie are the:

    a. meats
    b. vegetables
    c. fruits
    d. grains

19. The most energy-rich of the nutrients is:

    a. carbohydrate
    b. protein
    c. fat
    d. alcohol

Application Level Items:

20. You are explaining to a friend the characteristics of the most healthful diet based on the Dietary Guidelines. Which of the following would you include in your explanation?

    a. low in cholesterol
    b. moderate in sugar
    c. moderate in saturated fat
    d. a and b
    e. a and c

21. One of your best friends makes the statement that eggs are a bad food. Which of the following would be the best response to this statement?

    a. yes they are because they have a lot of cholesterol
    b. no they are not because they provide high quality protein
    c. yes they are because they cause heart disease
    d. they are neither good nor bad depending on how they are used in the total diet

22. How many calories are contained in a food that has 20 grams of carbohydrate, 15 grams of protein, and 8 grams of fat?

    a. 145
    b. 195
    c. 212
    d. 245

23. A food contains 8 grams of fat and a total of 212 calories. What percentage of the calories in the food come from fat?

    a. 25%
    b. 34%
    c. 46%
    d. 52%

24. An individual consumes a total of 3000 calories and 100 grams of fat in a day. Does this person's diet meet the goal of 30% or less calories from fat?

    a. yes
    b. no

25. Which of the following characteristics of a nutritious diet is illustrated by the statement that a certain amount of fiber in foods contributes to health of the digestive tract, but too much fiber leads to nutrient losses?

    a. moderation
    b. variety
    c. balance
    d. adequacy

ANSWERS

SUMMING UP

(1) food; (2) energy; (3) six; (4) organic; (5) water; (6) fats; (7) minerals; (8) essential; (9) nutrients; (10) growth; (11) brain; (12) nonnutrients; (13) experiments; (14) duplicated; (15) culture; (16) foodways; (17) social; (18) nutritional; (19) staple; (20) Healthy People; (21) monitoring; (22) variety; (23) calories; (24) adequacy; (25) moderation

CHAPTER GLOSSARY

Matching Exercise 1: (1) c; (2) i; (3) l; (4) n; (5) b; (6) f; (7) j; (8) a; (9) h; (10) m; (11) e; (12) k; (13) g; (14) d; (15) o
Matching Exercise 2: (1) g; (2) c; (3) l; (4) n; (5) b; (6) i; (7) e; (8) j; (9) m; (10) a; (11) f; (12) k; (13) d; (14) h

EXERCISES

Chapter Study Questions:

1. Protein can yield energy, but it also provides materials that form structures and working parts of body tissues.

2. Essential nutrients are those that the body cannot make for itself from other raw materials; they are the nutrients obtained in food and needed by the body; without them you will develop deficiencies.

3. Foods are thought to convey emotional satisfaction and hormonal stimuli that contribute to health; also they provide nonnutrients and other compounds that give them their tastes, aromas, colors, and other characteristics.

4. One reason is that some less well-known nutrients and some nonnutrients could be important to health and some foods may be better sources of these than others. Another reason is that a monotonous diet may deliver large amounts of toxins or contaminants.

5. The food industry offers thousands of foods, many of which are processed mixtures of the basic ones, and some of which are constructed mostly from artificial ingredients.

Short Answer Questions:

1. (a) carbohydrate; (b) fat; (c) protein; (d) vitamins

2. (a) water; (b) carbohydrate; (c) fat; (d) protein; (e) vitamins; (f) minerals

3. (a) carbohydrates; (b) fats; (c) protein

4. (a) personal preference; (b) habit; (c) ethnic heritage; (d) social pressure, (e) availability; (f) convenience; (g) economy; (h) positive associations; (i) emotional comfort; (j) values or beliefs; (k) nutritional value; (l) region of the country; (m) weight; (n) advertising

5. (a) adequacy; (b) balance; (c) calorie control, (d) moderation; (e) variety

Problem-Solving:

(1) b; (2) e; (3) c; (4) f; (5) a; (6) g; (7) d

Controversy Questions:

1. The work must survive a screening review by peers of scientists.

2. Membership in the American Society for Clinical Nutrition

3. An organization that awards meaningless degrees without requiring its students to meet educational standards.

4. Completion of a two-year academic degree from an accredited college or university and an approved dietetic technician program.

5. Administrative, clinical and nutrition support.

SAMPLE TEST ITEMS

1. c (p. 14-15)
2. a (p. 5)
3. d (p. 4)
4. b (p. 4)
5. c (p. 5)
6. e (p. 5)
7. d (p. 5-6)
8. a (p. 3)

9. d (p. 4)
10. b (p. 16)
11. c (p. 15)
12. a (p. 7)
13. d (p. 7)
14. b (p. 8)
15. c (p. 8-9)
16. c (p. 20-21)

17. a (p. 18-21)
18. b (p. 20)
19. c (p. 5)
20. d (p. 12)
21. d (p. 20-21)
22. c (p. 5)
23. b (p. 5)
24. a (p. 5)
25. a (p. 9)

CHAPTER 2

Nutrition Tools - Standards and Guidelines

CHAPTER OBJECTIVES

After completing this chapter, you should be able to:

1. Describe the roles *Dietary Reference Intakes (DRI)* and *Daily Values* play in achieving adequate nutrient intakes.

2. Describe how *Dietary Reference Intake* values are established for nutrients.

3. Recognize that many nations and international groups have published sets of standards similar to the DRI.

4. List the American College of Sports Medicine's recommendations for physical activity.

5. Identify the components of the *Daily Food Guide* and the *Food Guide Pyramid* and discuss how they are used to plan healthy diets.

6. Explain how exchange systems are useful to diet planners.

7. Discuss how consumers can use the ingredients list, nutrition facts panel, and health messages on food labels to make healthy food choices.

8. Describe possible actions of phytochemicals and functional foods and the evidence supporting their role in fighting certain diseases. (Controversy 2)

KEY CONCEPTS

✓ The Dietary Reference Intakes (DRI) are nutrient intake standards set for people living in the United States and Canada. The Daily Values are U.S. standards used on food labels.

✓ The DRI provide nutrient intake goals for individuals, provide a set of standards for researchers and makers of public policy, establish tolerable upper limits for nutrients that can be toxic in excess, and take into account new research on disease prevention. The DRI are composed of the RDA, AI, UL and EAR lists of values. The Daily Values are nutrient intake standards used on food labels.

✓ The DRI represent up-to-date, optimal, and safe nutrient intakes for healthy people in the United States and Canada.

✓ The DRI are based on scientific data and are designed to cover the needs of virtually all healthy people in the United States and Canada.

✓ The Daily Values are standards used on food labels to enable consumers to compare the nutrient values among foods.

✓ Many nations and groups issue recommendations for nutrient and energy intakes appropriate for specific groups of people.

✓ The Daily Food Guide sorts foods into groups based on their nutrients and origins. Then the plans suggest patterns of intake by group that will cover nutrient needs of adults.

✓ The Daily Food Guide and its visual image, the Food Guide Pyramid, convey the basics of planning a diet adequate in nutrients. The Food Guide Pyramid fails to show how to use nutrient-dense foods to form the bulk of food selections from each food group.

✓ Exchange lists facilitate calorie control by providing an understanding of how much carbohydrate, fat, and protein are in each food group.

✓ The Daily Food Guide specifies how many servings of foods from each group people need to consume to meet their nutrient requirements.

✓ A person wishing to avoid overconsuming calories must pay attention to serving sizes.

SUMMING UP

A committee of qualified nutrition experts from the United States and (1)_____ is

currently developing nutrient intake recommendations known as the (2) _____.

These recommendations are estimates of the needs of (3)_____ persons and are

intended to be used to plan diets for (4) _____. These recommended intakes take

into account (5) _____ as well as nutrient adequacy. Other values established

by the DRI Committee include (6) _____, which are used by researchers and

policy makers, and Tolerable Upper Intake Levels. The value for energy intake is set at the

(7)_____of the population's estimated energy requirements. Many nations and

international groups have published standards similar to the DRI. The (8) _____

recommendations are considered sufficient for the maintenance of health in nearly all healthy

people worldwide.

To help people plan menus, two kinds of planning tools are available including food

group plans and the (9) _____ system. The Daily Food Guide, and its visual

representation, the (10) _____, is based on five groups. The food groups are

represented in a pyramid-shape with (11) _____ at the bottom, indicating that

you should eat more of these foods than anything else. Fats, oils, and (12) _____

occupy the top of the pyramid, indicating they should be used sparingly. Exchange systems are

useful for those wishing to control (13) _____, for those who must control

carbohydrate intakes, and those who should control their intake of (14) _____

and saturated fat. The lists organize foods according to their calories, carbohydrate, fat,

saturated fat and (15) _____ contents. The exchange system highlights a fact

that the Food Guide Pyramid overlooks, in that most foods provide more than just one

(16) _____ nutrient.

The Nutrition Education and Labeling Act of 1990 set the requirements for nutrition

labeling information. According to law, every packaged food must state the (17) _____

name of the product, the name and address of the manufacturer, the (18) _____ contents and the ingredients, in (19)_____ order of predominance by weight. The (20) _____ informs consumers of the nutrient contents of the food. In addition to food energy, the label must include total fat (with breakdown of saturated fat), cholesterol, sodium, total carbohydrate (including fiber and sugars), (21) _____, vitamins A and C, and the minerals (22) _____ and iron. Some claims about health are allowed on food labels as long as they meet a strict set of guidelines set forth by the (23) _____.

CHAPTER GLOSSARY

Matching Exercise:

_____ 1. requirement	a. a set of nutrient intake standards designed for use on U.S. food labels
_____ 2. food group plans	b. a concentrate that has been brought back to its original strength by the addition of water
_____ 3. Daily Values	c. the amount of a nutrient that will just prevent the development of specific deficiency sign
_____ 4. balance study	d. claims linking food constituents with disease states
_____ 5. Nutrition Facts	e. diet planning tools that sort foods into groups based on origin and nutrient content and then specify that people should eat certain minimum numbers of servings of foods from each group
_____ 6. health claims	
_____ 7. exchange system	f. a laboratory study in which a person is fed a controlled diet and the intake and excretion of a nutrient are measured
_____ 8. reconstituted	
_____ 9. Dietary Reference Intakes	g. the panel of nutrition information required to appear on almost every packaged food
_____ 10. nutrient claims	h. a diet planning tool that organizes foods with respect to their nutrient contents and calorie amounts
	i. claims using approved wording to make statements about the nutrient value of foods
	j. a set of four lists of values for the dietary nutrient intakes of healthy people in the United States and Canada

EXERCISES

Answer these chapter study questions:

1. Why is the value set for energy intake not generous?

2. Describe the goals the DRI committee had in mind when setting the DRI values.

3. Identify drawbacks to the Food Guide Pyramid.

4. What would be the advantage of using the Food Guide Pyramid in conjunction with Exchange Lists when planning a diet?

5. Explain why the DRI values are not used on food labels.

Complete these short answer questions:

1. The three main groups of the exchange system are:

    a.
    b.
    c.

2. DRI recommended intakes exist for _____ vitamins and _____ minerals.

3. Dietary Reference Intakes include these four lists of values:

    a.
    b.
    c.
    d.

4. The five groups in the Food Guide Pyramid include:

    a.
    b.
    c.
    d.
    e.

5. Food labels must provide the following information on the panel called *"Nutrition Facts."*

    a.   g.
    b.   h.
    c.   i.
    d.   j.
    e.   k.
    f.   l.

6. Identify the number of calories provided by 1 exchange in each of the following exchange lists.

   a. Vegetable   = _____ calories
   b. Starch   = _____ calories
   c. Nonfat milk   = _____ calories
   d. Fat   = _____ calories
   e. Fruit   = _____ calories
   f. Medium-fat meat   = _____ calories
   g. Low-fat milk   = _____ calories
   h. High-fat meat   = _____ calories
   i. Whole milk   = _____ calories
   j. Lean meat   = _____ calories

Solve these problems:

1. Use the menu below to complete sections a-d which follow:

MENU

Breakfast	Lunch	Dinner
1 hard boiled egg	2 tbsp. peanut butter	3 oz. hamburger
1 oz. cornflakes	1 tsp. jelly	hamburger bun
1 cup skim milk	2 slices bread	2 tsp. mayonnaise
½ grapefruit	1 apple	½ cup baked beans
	1 diet cola	1 cup yogurt

   a. Categorize the foods in the menu according to the Food Guide Pyramid:

Breads, Cereals, and Other Grain Products	Fruits	Vegetables	Meat, Poultry, Fish, and Alternates	Milk Yogurt, and Cheese

   b. Which foods were you unable to classify?

c. Evaluate the adequacy of the menu according to the Food Guide Pyramid by comparing the number of actual servings with the number of recommended servings for an older adult.

Food Group	Recommended Servings	Actual Servings
Breads, cereals, and other grain products	6	_____
Fruits	2	_____
Vegetables	3	_____
Meat, poultry, fish, and alternates	2	_____
Milk, yogurt, and cheese	2-3	_____

d. Categorize the foods in the menu into exchanges by placing an X in the appropriate blank.

	Starch	Meats	Vegetables	Fruits	Milks	Fats	Other
egg	___	___	___	___	___	___	___
cornflakes	___	___	___	___	___	___	___
skim milk	___	___	___	___	___	___	___
jelly	___	___	___	___	___	___	___
grapefruit	___	___	___	___	___	___	___
peanut butter	___	___	___	___	___	___	___
bread	___	___	___	___	___	___	___
apple	___	___	___	___	___	___	___
diet cola	___	___	___	___	___	___	___
hamburger	___	___	___	___	___	___	___
bun	___	___	___	___	___	___	___
mayonnaise	___	___	___	___	___	___	___
baked beans	___	___	___	___	___	___	___
yogurt	___	___	___	___	___	___	___

2. a. How many calories are in a day's meal which provides 260 grams carbohydrate, 30 grams protein, and 60 grams of fat? _____ calories

b. What percent of the calories are from carbohydrate? _____ %

c. What percent of the calories are from fat? _____ %

d. How does the percentage of calories from fat compare to the amount in the *Healthy People 2010 Objectives?*

Solve these controversy questions:

1. What advice would you give someone who looks to consume chocolate to reduce the risk of heart attack and stroke?

2. Why do food manufacturers often refine away the natural flavonoids in foods?

3. What are some foods common to many Asian diets that contain phytosterols?

4. Which types of cancer occur less frequently in people who consume five tomato-containing meals per week?

5. What are probiotics?

STUDY AIDS

Use the following table and figure in your textbook as study aids: Table 2-3 on page 42; Figure 2-4 on pages 36-37.

SAMPLE TEST ITEMS

Comprehension Level Items:

1. Recommendations for dietary nutrient intakes of healthy people in the United States and Canada are called:

   a. Recommended Nutrient Intakes
   b. Daily Values
   c. Adequate Intakes
   d. Dietary Reference Intakes
   e. Tolerable Upper Intake Levels

2. Which of the following establishes population-wide average requirements that researchers and policy makers use in their work?

   a. Adequate Intakes
   b. Tolerable Upper Intake Limits
   c. Estimated Average Requirements
   d. Recommended Dietary Allowances

3. All of the following adjectives are descriptive of the Dietary Reference Intakes *except:*

   a. minimal
   b. approximate
   c. recommendations
   d. generous

4. The value set for energy is set at the average of the population's estimated energy requirements in order to:

   a. compensate for lack of physical activity
   b. discourage overconsumption of energy which would lead to obesity
   c. encourage a decrease in fat consumption
   d. ensure generous allowances of fat and carbohydrate

5. The term *Daily Values* appears on:

   a. fresh meats
   b. refined foods
   c. food labels
   d. fresh vegetables

6. In the Food Guide Pyramid, all of the following foods are grouped together at the top of the pyramid **_except_**:

   a. fruit rolls
   b. doughnuts
   c. salad dressing
   d. cream

7. In the Food Guide Pyramid, potatoes are included in the _____ group.

   a. milk
   b. fruit
   c. meat
   d. vegetable

8. In the food exchange lists, all of the food portions on one list have about the same number of calories and about the same amount of energy nutrients.

   a. true
   b. false

9. In the exchange lists, 1/2 cup of any cooked vegetable in the vegetable exchange list provides about _____ calories.

   a. 25
   b. 45
   c. 60
   d. 80

10. In the exchange lists, meats and substitutes are separated into _____ categories, based on fat content.

    a. two
    b. three
    c. four
    d. five

11. Corn and potatoes are listed in the _____ list of the exchange system.

    a. meats
    b. vegetables
    c. starch
    d. fat

12. The exchange system highlights the fact that most foods provide more than one energy nutrient.

    a. true
    b. false

13. Based on the Food Guide Pyramid, people should consume a minimum of _____ servings from the bread and cereals group each day.

    a. two
    b. four
    c. five
    d. six

14. Which of the following is **_not_** a drawback of the Food Guide Pyramid?

    a. it is very rigid and difficult to use
    b. it fails to limit food choices to foods low in calories
    c. it is difficult to identify high-fat foods within a group
    d. it can lead to consistently nutrient-poor choices

15. The American College of Sports Medicine recommends exercise for a duration of at least 30 minutes total daily.

    a. true
    b. false

16. Which of the following is the major purpose of the Daily Values listed on food labels?

    a. prevent chronic diseases
    b. allow comparisons among foods
    c. discourage overconsumption of calories
    d. prevent nutrient toxicity

17. A food with *Healthy* as part of its name cannot contain any nutrient or food constituent in an amount known to increase disease risk.

    a. true
    b. false

18. Which of the following nutrient information is **_not_** required on food labels?

    a. fat in grams per serving
    b. polyunsaturated fat in grams per serving
    c. saturated fat in grams per serving
    d. cholesterol in milligrams per serving

19. Which of the following health claims relating the roles of nutrients and food constituents to disease states is *not* allowable under FDA guidelines?

    a. calcium as related to osteoporosis
    b. sodium as related to hypertension
    c. dietary fat as related to cancer
    d. grains, fruits and vegetables as related to cancer
    e. sodium as related to coronary heart disease

20. According to current food labeling laws, whole milk cannot make a claim about osteoporosis because it contains too much saturated fat.

    a. true
    b. false

Application Level Items:

21. Which of the following in *not* one of the criteria used for establishing serving sizes found in the Food Guide Pyramid?

    a. an amount of food typically consumed at one sitting
    b. an amount typically served in restaurants
    c. an amount of food that delivers a known quantity of key nutrients
    d. an amount of food used in previous food guides to describe a serving

22. How many calories are contained in the following meal pattern for a lunch meal: 1 lean meat, 1 starch, 1 vegetable, 1 fruit, and 1 fat?

    a. 235
    b. 256
    c. 265
    d. 300

23. An ingredient list states that a food product contains peas, water, carrots, sugar, and salt. Which of these ingredients is present in the smallest quantity?

    a. peas
    b. carrots
    c. sugar
    d. salt
    e. water

24. You see the following ingredient list on a cereal label: *wheat, sugar, raisins, brown sugar, syrup, and salt.* You therefore conclude that this product:

    a. is a good source of fiber
    b. contains 100% whole wheat
    c. is a nutritious food choice
    d. contains close to half its weight in sugar

25. The Nutrition Facts Panel on a box of cereal lists the following information for amounts per serving: **167** *calories; 27 calories from fat; 3 g total fat.* What percentage of the calories are provided by fat?

    a. 3%
    b. 11%
    c. 16%
    d. 27%

ANSWERS

SUMMING UP

(1) Canada; (2) Dietary Reference Intakes; (3) healthy; (4) individuals; (5) disease prevention; (6) Estimated Average Requirements; (7) average; (8) WHO/FAO; (9) exchange; (10) Food Guide Pyramid; (11) grains; (12) sweets;(13) calories; (14) fat; (15) protein; (16) energy; (17) common; (18) net; (19) descending; (20) Nutrition Facts Panel; (21) protein; (22) calcium; (23) Food and Drug Administration

CHAPTER GLOSSARY

Matching Exercise: (1) c; (2) e; (3) a; (4) f; (5) g; (6) d; (7) h; (8) b; (9) j; (10) i.

EXERCISES

Chapter Study Questions:

1. Because too much energy is bad for health and leads to obesity, while too little energy may cause undernutrition.

2. The four goals of the committee included setting intake recommendations for individuals, preventing chronic diseases, facilitating nutrition research and policy, and establishing safety guidelines.

3. The Food Guide Pyramid does not limit choices to foods low in calories. It is difficult to identify high-fat and high-sugar foods within a group by using the Food Guide Pyramid. Finally, a person may follow all of the Guide's rules and still make consistently nutrient-poor food choices and fail to meet the day's needs for some nutrients.

4. The Food Guide Pyramid provides the framework that ensures nutrient adequacy while the Exchange Lists facilitate calorie control by providing an understanding of where the carbohydrates, fats, and proteins are in foods.

5. The DRI values vary from group to group, whereas on a food label, one set of values must apply to everyone. Also, the label must specify daily amounts of food constituents not yet covered by the DRI, such as fat, carbohydrate and fiber.

Short Answer Questions:

1. (a) carbohydrate group; (b) fat group; (c) meat and meat substitutes group

2. 14; 12

3. (a) Recommended Dietary Allowances; (b) Adequate Intakes; (c) Tolerable Upper Intake Levels; (d) Estimated Average Requirements

4. (a) bread, cereal, rice and pasta; (b) fruits; (c) vegetables; (d) meat, poultry, fish, dry beans, eggs and nuts; (e) milk, yogurt and cheese

5. (a) serving size; (b) servings per container; (c) calories from fat; (d) fat grams per serving including saturated fat; (e) cholesterol; (f) sodium; (g) total carbohydrate including fiber and sugars; (h) protein; (i) vitamin A; (j) vitamin C; (k) calcium; (l) iron

6. (a) 25; (b) 80; (c) 90; (d) 45; (e) 60; (f) 75; (g) 120; (h) 100; (i) 150; (j) 55

Problem-Solving:

1. a.

Breads, Cereals, and Other Grain Products	Fruits	Vegetables	Meat, Poultry, Fish, and Alternates	Milk Yogurt, and Cheese
cornflakes bread hamburger bun	grapefruit apple		egg peanut butter hamburger baked beans	skim milk yogurt

    b. jelly; diet cola; mayonnaise

    c. breads, cereals, and other grain products - 5 servings
       fruits - 2 servings
       vegetables - 0 servings
       meat, poultry, fish, and alternates - 4 servings
       milk, yogurt, and cheese - 2 servings

d.

	Starch	Meats	Vegetables	Fruits	Milks	Fats	Other
egg		X					
cornflakes	X						
skim milk					X		
jelly							X
grapefruit				X			
peanut butter		X				X	
bread	X						
apple				X			
diet cola							X
hamburger		X					
bun	X						
mayonnaise						X	
baked beans	X						
yogurt					X		

2. (a) 1700 calories; (b) 61 % calories from carbohydrate; (c) 32% calories from fat; (d) the percent calories from fat is above the recommended level of 30%

Controversy Questions:

1. It would be better to obtain flavonoids from nutrient-dense food sources such as fruits, vegetables or green or black tea because chocolate promotes weight gain and contributes fat and sugar to the diet.

2. Because they impart a bitter taste to foods and most consumers desire milder flavors.

3. Soybeans and their products including tofu, miso and soy drink

4. Cancers of the esophagus, prostate and stomach

5. Probiotics are microorganisms believed to alter the native bacteria colonies in the body in ways that may reduce diseases.

SAMPLE TEST ITEMS

1. d (p. 30)
2. c (p. 31)
3. a (p. 32-33)
4. b (p. 34)
5. c (p. 34)
6. b (p. 36-37)
7. d (p. 36)
8. a (p. 39)
9. a (Appendix D)

10. c (Appendix D)
11. c (Appendix D)
12. a (p. 39)
13. d (p. 38)
14. a (p. 38-39)
15. a (p. 35)
16. b (p. 34)
17. a (p. 49)

18. b (p. 46)
19. e (p. 48)
20. a (p. 49)
21. b (p. 42)
22. c (Appendix D)
23. d (p. 46)
24. d (p. 46-47)
25. c (p. 47)

CHAPTER 3

The Remarkable Body

CHAPTER OBJECTIVES

After completing this chapter, you should be able to:

1. Identify the basic needs of cells and describe how cells are organized into tissues, organs, and systems.

2. Describe the major functions of the cardiovascular, hormonal, nervous, digestive, and excretory systems.

3. Describe the mechanical and chemical digestive processes in order of their occurrence in the body.

4. Differentiate between the mechanical and chemical aspects of digestion.

5. Discuss the processes of absorption, transportation, and storage of nutrients.

6. Describe alcohol's effects on the body and whether the benefits of alcohol outweigh the risks. (Controversy 3)

KEY CONCEPTS

✓ The body's cells need energy, oxygen, and nutrients, including water, to remain healthy and do their work. Genes direct the making of each cell's machinery, including enzymes. Specialized cells are grouped together to form tissues and organs; organs work together in body systems.

✓ Blood and lymph deliver nutrients to all the body's cells and carry waste materials away from them. Blood also delivers oxygen to cells. The cardiovascular system ensures that these fluids circulate properly among all organs.

✓ Glands secrete hormones that act as messengers to help regulate body processes.

✓ The nervous system joins the hormonal system to regulate body processes through communication among all the organs. Together, the hormonal and nervous systems respond to the need for food, govern the act of eating, regulate digestion, and call for the stress response.

✓ The immune system enables the body to resist disease.

✓ The preference for sweet, salty, and fatty tastes seems to be inborn and can lead to over consumption of foods that offer them.

✓ The digestive tract is a flexible, muscular tube that digests food and absorbs its nutrients and some nonnutrients.

✓ The digestive tract moves food through its various processing chambers by mechanical means. The mechanical actions include chewing, mixing by the stomach, adding fluid, and moving the tract's contents by peristalsis. After digestion and absorption, wastes are excreted.

✓ Chemical digestion begins in the mouth, where food is mixed with an enzyme in saliva that acts on carbohydrates. Digestion continues in the stomach, where stomach enzymes and acid break down protein. Digestion then continues in the small intestine; there the liver and gallbladder contribute bile that emulsifies fat, and the pancreas and small intestine donate enzymes that continue digestion so that absorption can occur.

✓ The healthy digestive system is capable of adjusting to almost any diet and can handle any combination of foods with ease.

✓ The mechanical and chemical actions of the digestive tract break foods down to nutrients, and large nutrients to their smaller building blocks, with remarkable efficiency.

✓ The digestive system feeds the rest of the body and is itself sensitive to malnutrition. The folds and villi of the small intestine enlarge its surface area to facilitate nutrient absorption through countless cells to the blood and lymph. These transport systems then deliver the nutrients to all the body cells.

✓ The digestive tract has many ways to communicate its needs. By taking the time to listen, you will obtain a complete understanding of the mechanics of the digestive tract and its signals.

✓ The kidneys adjust the blood's composition in response to the body's needs, disposing of everyday wastes and helping remove toxins. Nutrients, including water, and exercise help keep the kidneys healthy.

✓ The body's energy stores are of two principal kinds: fat in fat cells (in potentially large quantities) and glycogen in muscle and liver cells (in smaller quantities). Other tissues store other nutrients.

✓ To achieve optimal function, the body's systems require nutrients from outside. These have to be supplied through a human being's conscious food choices.

SUMMING UP

The body is composed of trillions of (1) _____ and the nature of their work is determined by genes. Among the cells' most basic needs are (2) _____,

oxygen, and nutrients to remain healthy and do their work. Specialized cells are grouped together to form tissues and (3) _____ . Body (4) _____ supply the tissues continuously with energy, oxygen and nutrients. The body's main fluids are the blood and

(5) _____. Blood travels within the arteries, (6)_____ and capillaries, as well as within the heart's chambers.

As the blood travels through the cardiovascular system, it picks up oxygen in the

(7) _____and also releases carbon dioxide there. As it passes through the digestive system, the blood picks up most (8) _____, other than fats, for distribution elsewhere. All blood leaving the digestive system is routed directly to the (9) _____. The blood is cleansed of its wastes as it passes through the (10) _____.

The hormonal and (11) _____- systems regulate body processes through communication among all the organs. They respond to the need for food, govern the act of eating, regulate (12) _____ and call for the stress response. The (13) _____ system's job is to digest food to its component nutrients and then to (14) _____ those nutrients, leaving behind the substances that are appropriate to excrete. To do this, the system works at two levels, one mechanical and the other (15) _____.

The body's cells need nutrients around the (16) _____ which requires systems of (17) _____ and release to meet the cells' needs between meals. However,

34

some (18) _____ are stored in the body in much larger quantities than others. The

liver converts excess energy-containing nutrients into two forms, glycogen and

(19) _____ . Body stores for other nutrients include the liver and fat cells which

store many vitamins and the (20) _____ which provides reserves of calcium,

sodium, and other minerals.

CHAPTER GLOSSARY

Matching Exercise 1:

_____ 1. capillaries	a.	a group of related organs that work together to perform a function
_____ 2. fat cells	b.	systems of cells working together to perform specialized tasks
_____ 3. body system	c.	units of a cell's inheritance, made of the chemical DNA (deoxyribonucleic acid)
_____ 4. hormones	d.	a part of the brain that senses a variety of conditions in the blood, such as temperature, glucose content, salt content, and others
_____ 5. glucagon		
_____ 6. enzyme	e.	a protein that promotes a chemical reaction
	f.	cells that specialize in the storage of fat and that form the fat tissue
_____ 7. cells	g.	the wave-like muscular squeezing of the esophagus, stomach, and small intestine that pushes their contents along
_____ 8. tissues	h.	discrete structural units made of tissues that perform specific jobs, such as the heart, liver, and brain
_____ 9. arteries	i.	chemicals that are secreted by glands into the blood in response to conditions in the body that require regulation
_____ 10. absorb	j.	the major hormone that elicits the stress response
	k.	blood vessels that carry blood containing fresh oxygen supplies from the heart to the tissues
_____ 11. organs	l.	minute, weblike blood vessels that connect arteries to veins and permit transfer of materials between blood and tissues
_____ 12. genes	m.	the body's instinctive hormone- and nerve-mediated reaction to danger
_____ 13. peristalsis	n.	a hormone from the pancreas that stimulates the liver to release glucose into the bloodstream
_____ 14. fight-or-flight reaction	o.	to take in, as nutrients are taken into the intestinal cells after digestion; the main function of the digestive tract with respect to nutrients
_____ 15. hypothalamus	p.	the smallest units in which independent life can exist
_____ 16. insulin	q.	a hormone from the pancreas that helps glucose enter cells from the blood
_____ 17. epinephrine		

Matching Exercise 2:

_____ 1. lungs

_____ 2. nephrons

_____ 3. mucus

_____ 4. gastric juice

_____ 5. extracellular fluid

_____ 6. pancreatic juice

_____ 7. emulsifier

_____ 8. pH

_____ 9. chyme

_____ 10. bile

_____ 11. diarrhea

_____ 12. lymph

_____ 13. bicarbonate

_____ 14. plasma

_____ 15. colon

_____ 16. feces

_____ 17. villi

_____ 18. stomach

a. fluid residing outside the cells

b. the body's organs of gas exchange

c. the fluid that moves from the bloodstream into tissue spaces and then travels in its own vessels, which eventually drain back into the bloodstream

d. waste material remaining after digestion and absorption are complete

e. a measure of acidity on a point scale

f. the large intestine

g. a slippery coating of the digestive tract lining (and other body linings) that protect the cells from exposure to digestive juices (and other destructive agents)

h. a compound made by the liver, stored in the gallbladder, and released into the small intestine when needed

i. fluid secreted by the pancreas that contains enzymes to digest carbohydrate, fat, and protein as well as sodium bicarbonate, a neutralizing agent

j. fingerlike projections of the sheets of cells that line the intestinal tract

k. frequent, watery bowel movements usually caused by diet, stress, or irritation of the colon

l. the working units in the kidneys, consisting of intermeshed blood vessels and tubules

m. the cell-free fluid part of blood and lymph

n. muscular, elastic, pouchlike organ of the digestive tract that grinds and churns swallowed food and mixes it with acid and enzymes, forming chyme

o. the fluid resulting from the actions of the stomach upon a meal

p. the digestive secretion of the stomach

q. a compound with both water-soluble and fat-soluble portions that can attract fats and oils into water to form an emulsion

r. a common alkaline chemical; a secretion of the pancreas

Matching Exercise 3:

_____ 1. kidneys

_____ 2. liver

_____ 3. digest

_____ 4. cortex

_____ 5. intestine

_____ 6. norepinephrine

_____ 7. veins

_____ 8. digestive system

_____ 9. blood

_____ 10. large intestine

_____ 11. heartburn

_____ 12. pyloric valve

_____ 13. hernia

_____ 14. constipation

_____ 15. small intestine

_____ 16. sphincter

_____ 17. bladder

a. to break molecules into smaller molecules; a main function of the digestive tract with respect to food

b. the fluid of the cardiovascular system composed of water, red. and white blood cells, other formed particles, nutrients, oxygen, and other constituents

c. the outermost layer of something

d. blood vessels that carry blood, with the carbon dioxide it has collected, from the tissues back to the heart

e. a compound related to epinephrine that helps to elicit the stress response

f. a pair of organs that filter wastes from the blood, make urine, and release it to the bladder for excretion from the body

g. a large, lobed organ that lies just under the ribs

h. a long, tubular organ of digestion and the site of nutrient absorption

i. the body system composed of organs that break down complex food particles into smaller, absorbable products

j. the portion of the intestine that completes the absorption process

k. the circular muscle of the lower stomach that regulates the flow of partly digested food into the small intestine

l. a 20-foot length of small-diameter intestine that is the major site of digestion of food and absorption of nutrients

m. infrequent, difficult bowel movements often caused by diet, inactivity, dehydration, or medication

n. a protrusion of an organ or part of an organ through the wall of the body chamber that normally contains the organ

o. a burning sensation in the chest (heart) area caused by backflow of stomach acid into the esophagus

p. a circular muscle surrounding, and able to close, a body opening

q. the sac that holds urine until time for elimination

Matching Exercise 4:

_____ 1. antibodies

_____ 2. metabolism

_____ 3. immune system

_____ 4. microbes

_____ 5. antigen

_____ 6. lymphocytes

_____ 7. pancreas

_____ 8. neurotransmitters

_____ 9. microvilli

_____ 10. phagocytes

_____ 11. hiccups

_____ 12. T-cells

_____ 13. irritable bowel syndrome

_____ 14. ulcer

_____ 15. B-cells

_____ 16. gastro-esophageal reflux disease

_____ 17. antacids

_____ 18. glycogen

a. lymphocytes that attack antigens

b. a system of tissues and organs that defend the body against antigens, foreign materials that have penetrated the skin or body linings

c. the sum of all physical and chemical changes taking place in living cells

d. intermittent disturbance of bowel function, especially diarrhea or alternating diarrhea and constipation

e. chemicals that are released at the end of a nerve cell when a nerve impulse arrives

f. proteins, made by cells of the immune system, that are expressly designed to combine with and to inactivate specific antigens

g. bacteria, viruses, or other organisms invisible to the naked eye, some of which cause diseases

h. medications that react directly and immediately with the acid of the stomach, neutralizing it

i. spasms of both the vocal cords and the diaphragm, causing periodic, audible, short, inhaled coughs

j. a microbe or substance that is foreign to the body

k. white blood cells that can ingest and destroy antigens

l. white blood cells that participate in the immune response; B-cells and T-cells

m. lymphocytes that produce antibodies

n. a severe and chronic splashing of stomach acid and enzymes into the esophagus, throat, mouth, or airway that causes inflammation and injury to those organs

o. a storage form of carbohydrate energy

p. tiny, hairlike projections on each cell of every villus that can trap nutrient particles and transport them into the cells

q. an organ with two main functions; one is an endocrine function and the other is an exocrine function

r. an erosion in the topmost, and sometimes underlying, layers of cells that form a lining

EXERCISES

Answer these chapter study questions:

1. Identify and describe three factors necessary to ensure efficient circulation of fluid to all body cells.

2. Differentiate between the functions of glands and hormones.

3. Differentiate between the mechanical aspect of digestion and the chemical aspect of digestion.

4. Describe how the body's digestive system is affected by:

   a. severe undernutrition

   b. lack of dietary fiber

5. What is the difference between glycogen and fat?

Complete these short answer questions:

1. The cells most basic needs include:

    a.
    b.
    c.

2. The body's main fluids are the _____ and _____.

3. These are the central controllers of the nervous system:

    a.
    b.

4. The body's hormonal balance is altered by:

    a.
    b.
    c.

5. Five factors required to support the health of the kidneys include:

    a.
    b.
    c.
    d.
    e.

6. The liver converts excess energy containing nutrients into two forms including _____ and _____.

Solve these problems:

For questions 1-8, match the organs of the digestive system, listed on the left, to their primary functions, listed on the right.

_____ 1. stomach

_____ 2. liver

_____ 3. large intestine

_____ 4. mouth

_____ 5. pancreas

_____ 6. esophagus

_____ 7. small intestine

_____ 8. gallbladder

a.   manufactures enzymes to digest all energy-producing nutrients and releases bicarbonate to neutralize stomach acid

b.   stores bile until needed

c.   churns, mixes, and grinds food to a liquid mass

d.   passes food to the stomach

e.   manufactures bile to help digest fats

f.   reabsorbs water and minerals

g.   secretes enzymes that digest carbohydrate, fat, and protein; absorbs nutrients

h.   chews food and mixes it with saliva

Solve these controversy questions:

1.   Why is the term moderation difficult to define in relationship to alcohol consumption?

2.   How does food slow the absorption of alcohol?

3. What advice would you give someone who wants to drink alcohol socially but not become intoxicated?

4. Why are nutrient deficiencies an inevitable consequence of alcohol abuse?

5. What components of red wine are thought to be related to its health promoting qualities?

STUDY AID

Use the following table in your textbook as a study aid: Table 3-1 on page 82.

SAMPLE TEST ITEMS

Comprehension Level Items:

1. Genes direct the making of a piece of protein machinery which is most often a (an):

    a. antibody
    b. hormone
    c. enzyme
    d. antigen

2. Every cell continuously uses up:

   a. oxygen
   b. nutrients
   c. carbon dioxide
   d. a and b
   e. b and c

3. All blood leaving the digestive system is routed directly to the:

   a. pancreas
   b. liver
   c. kidneys
   d. gallbladder

4. The blood often serves as an indicator of disorders caused by dietary deficiencies or imbalances of vitamins and minerals.

   a. true
   b. false

5. Hormones act as messengers that stimulate various organs to take appropriate actions.

   a. true
   b. false

6. When the pancreas detects a high concentration of the blood's sugar, glucose, it:

   a. secretes a hormone called glucagon
   b. stimulates the liver to release glucose into the blood
   c. stimulates special nerve cells in the hypothalamus
   d. releases a hormone called insulin

7. Which of the following statements is *not* true concerning the hormonal system?

   a. it regulates the menstrual cycle in women
   b. it helps to regulate hunger and appetite
   c. it is affected by nutrition very little
   d. it regulates the body's reaction to stress

8. Which of the following occur(s) as part of the stress response?

   a. the pupils of the eyes widen
   b. the heart races to rush oxygen to the muscles
   c. the digestive system speeds up
   d. a and b
   e. a and c

9. The mechanical job of digestion is to:

   a. chew and crush foods
   b. add fluid
   c. secrete enzymes
   d. a and c
   e. a and b

10. The major site for digestion of food and absorption of nutrients is the:

    a. small intestine
    b. colon
    c. stomach
    d. liver

11. Which of the following ensures that the digestive tract lining will **not** be digested?

    a. enzymes
    b. mucus
    c. bile
    d. hydrochloric acid

For questions 12-16, match the digestive organs, listed on the left, with their appropriate functions, listed on the right.

_____12. small intestine

_____13. stomach

_____14. pancreas

_____15. large intestine

_____16. anus

   a. releases bicarbonate to neutralize stomach acid
   b. churns, mixes, and grinds food to a liquid mass
   c. cells of wall absorb nutrients into blood and lymph
   d. passes any unabsorbed nutrients, waste (fiber, bacteria), and some water to rectum
   e. manufactures bile to help digest fats
   f. holds rectum closed

17. Which of the following is(are) the main task(s) of the colon?

    a. to absorb fiber
    b. to reabsorb water
    c. to absorb some minerals
    d. a and b
    e. b and c

18. The digestive tract can adjust to whatever mixture of foods is presented to it.

    a. true
    b. false

19. Characteristics of the cells of the intestinal lining include:

    a. they are very efficient
    b. they are selective
    c. they are inefficient
    d. a and b
    e. b and c

20. Which of the following nutrients should be consumed in intervals throughout the day based on the body's storage systems?

    a. fat
    b. carbohydrate
    c. sodium
    d. protein

Application Level Items:

21. Why does all blood first circulate to the lungs and then return to the heart?

    a. in order to provide all tissues with oxygenated blood fresh from the lungs
    b. to deliver needed nutrients to the heart after disposing of carbon dioxide in the lungs
    c. to receive impetus from heartbeats that push blood out to all other body tissues
    d. a and b
    e. a and c

22. To avoid constipation you would:

    a. choose foods that provide enough fiber
    b. drink enough water
    c. change your diet quickly
    d. a and b
    e. b and c

23. In a healthy individual, blood glucose levels are maintained by:

    a. glands
    b. enzymes
    c. hormones
    d. a and b
    e. a and c

24. Gurgling noises from the digestive tract are most likely the result of:

    a. consuming too many high fiber foods
    b. gulping air with each swallow of food
    c. eating too much food at one time
    d. failing to relax after eating

25. Which of the following would you recommend for someone complaining about heartburn?

    a. suggest that he/she take antacids to neutralize the acid
    b. suggest that he/she drink milk to coat the lining of the stomach
    c. suggest that he/she avoid irritating foods and lay down after meals
    d. suggest that he/she eat smaller meals and drink liquids an hour before or after meals

26. Your friend tells you that she has problems digesting fruit and meat when she combines them in her diet. What would be your response?

    a. the digestive tract can't handle more than one task at a time
    b. meat and fruit should never be eaten in combination
    c. after eating fruit, wait at least three hours before consuming meat
    d. the digestive system can adjust to whatever mixture of foods is presented to it

ANSWERS

SUMMING UP

(1) cells; (2) energy; (3) organs; (4) fluids; (5) lymph; (6) veins; (7) lungs; (8) nutrients; (9) liver; (10) kidneys; (11) nervous; (12) digestion; (13) digestive; (14) absorb; (15) chemical; (16) clock; (17) storage; (18) nutrients; (19) fat; (20) bones

CHAPTER GLOSSARY

Matching Exercise 1: (1) l; (2) f; (3) a; (4) i; (5) n; (6) e; (7) p; (8) b; (9) k; (10) o; (11) h; (12) c; (13) g; (14) m; (15) d; (16) q; (17) j
Matching Exercise 2: (1) b; (2) l; (3) g; (4) p; (5) a; (6) i; (7) q; (8) e; (9) o; (10) h; (11) k; (12) c; (13) r; (14) m; (15) f; (16) d; (17) j; (18) n
Matching Exercise 3: (1) f; (2) g; (3) a; (4) c; (5) h; (6) e; (7) d; (8) i; (9) b; (10) j; (11) o; (12) k; (13) n; (14) m; (15) l; (16) p; (17) q
Matching Exercise 4: (1) f; (2) c; (3) b; (4) g; (5) j; (6) l; (7) q; (8) e; (9) p; (10) k; (11) i; (12) a; (13) d; (14) r; (15) m; (16) n; (17) h; (18) o

EXERCISES

Chapter Study Questions:

1. Drinking sufficient water to replace water lost each day; maintaining cardiovascular fitness, which requires attention to nutrition and physical activity; and healthy red blood cells because they carry oxygen to all other cells, enabling them to use fuels for energy.

2. Glands are organs that monitor conditions that need regulation and produce hormones to regulate those conditions. Hormones are chemicals that are secreted by glands into the blood in response to conditions in the body that require regulation.

3. The mechanical aspects of digestion include chewing, mixing by the stomach, adding fluid, and moving the digestive tract's contents by peristalsis. The chemical aspects of digestion involve several organs of the digestive system that secrete special digestive juices that contain enzymes that break nutrients down into their component parts.

4a. The absorptive surface of the small intestine shrinks and makes it impossible to obtain the few nutrients that the limited food supply may make available.

4b. The digestive tract muscles have too little undigested bulk to push against and get too little exercise, which make them become weak.

5. Glycogen is stored in the liver and the muscles and it is a storage form of carbohydrate energy. Fat is a storage form of lipid energy and is stored in the fat cells. Fat tissue has virtually unlimited storage capacity, but the liver can only store a limited supply of glycogen.

Short Answer Questions:

1. (a) energy; (b) oxygen; (c) essential nutrients

2. blood; lymph

3. (a) brain; (b) spinal cord

4. (a) fasting; (b) feeding; (c) exercise

5. (a) a strong cardiovascular system; (b) abundant water supply; (c) sufficient energy; (d) exercise; (e) vitamins and minerals

6. glycogen; fat

Problem-Solving:

(1) c; (2) e; (3) f; (4) h; (5) a; (6) d; (7) g; (8) b

Controversy Questions:

1. Because no single upper limit of alcohol per day is appropriate for everyone and tolerances to alcohol differ.

2. Alcohol in a stomach filled with food has a low probability of touching the walls of the stomach and diffusing through; food also holds alcohol in the stomach longer, slowing its entry into the highly absorptive small intestine.

3. The person should eat high carbohydrate snacks that slow absorption, and high fat snacks that slow peristalsis to keep the alcohol in the stomach longer. The person should also add water or ice to drinks to dilute them and choose non-alcoholic beverages first and then every other round to quench thirst.

4. Because alcohol displaces food and interferes directly with the body's use of nutrients by disrupting every tissue's metabolism of nutrients.

5. Wine has a high potassium content that may lower high blood pressure; wine facilitates the absorption of potassium, calcium, phosphorous, magnesium and zinc; wine also contains flavonoids that are antioxidants that may protect the cardiovascular system against damage from oxidation that leads to heart disease.

SAMPLE TEST ITEMS

1.	c (p. 69)	10.	a (p. 80)	19.	d (p. 83)
2.	d (p. 69)	11.	b (p. 80)	20.	b (p. 88)
3.	b (p. 71)	12.	c (p. 77)	21.	e (p. 69-71)
4.	a (p. 71)	13.	b (p. 77)	22.	d (p. 86)
5.	a (p. 72)	14.	a (p. 77)	23.	e (p. 72-73)
6.	d (p. 72)	15.	d (p. 77)	24.	b (p. 85)
7.	c (p. 73)	16.	f (p. 77)	25.	d (p. 85)
8.	d (p. 73)	17.	e (p. 79-80)	26.	d (p. 81)
9.	e (p. 77-79)	18.	a (p. 81)		

CHAPTER 4

The Carbohydrates: Sugar, Starch, Glycogen, and Fiber

CHAPTER OBJECTIVES

After completing this chapter, you should be able to:

1. Distinguish among the various carbohydrates found in foods and in the human body.

2. Describe the body's use of glucose to provide energy or to make glycogen and fat.

3. Discuss diabetes, hypoglycemia, and lactose intolerance and their relationship to carbohydrate intake.

4. Discuss the roles of fiber-rich foods in the maintenance of the body's health and identify foods rich in fiber.

5. Assess the role sugar and alternative sweeteners play in one's diet. (Controversy 4)

The Carbohydrates: Sugar, Starch, Glycogen, and Fiber

KEY CONCEPTS

✓ Through photosynthesis, plants combine carbon dioxide, water, and the sun's energy to form glucose. Carbohydrates are made of carbon, hydrogen, and oxygen held together by energy containing bonds: carbo means "carbon"; hydrate means "water."

✓ Glucose is the most important monosaccharide in the human body. Most other monosaccharides and disaccharides become glucose in the body.

✓ Starch is the storage form of glucose in plants and is also nutritive for human beings.

✓ Glycogen is the storage form of glucose in animals and human beings.

✓ Little fiber is digested by the enzymes in the human digestive tract. Much of the fiber passes through the digestive tract unchanged.

✓ Complex carbohydrates are the preferred energy source for the body.

✓ Fibers aid in maintaining the health of the digestive tract and help to prevent or control certain diseases. Most people need between 20 and 40 grams of fiber each day.

✓ Fiber needs are best met with whole foods. Purified fiber in large doses can have undesirable effects.

✓ With respect to starch and sugars, the main task of the various body systems is to convert them to glucose to fuel the cells' work. Fibers help regulate digestion and contribute a little energy.

✓ Lactose intolerance is a common condition in which the body fails to produce sufficient amounts of the enzyme needed to digest the sugar of milk. Uncomfortable symptoms result and can lead to milk avoidance. Lactose-intolerant people and those allergic to milk need milk alternatives that contain calcium.

✓ Without glucose, the body is forced to alter its use of protein and fats. The body breaks down its own muscles and other protein tissues to make glucose and converts its fats into ketone bodies, incurring ketosis.

✓ Glycogen is the body's form of stored glucose. The liver stores glycogen for use by the whole body. Muscles have their own private glycogen stock for their exclusive use. The hormone glucagon acts to liberate stored glucose from liver glycogen.

✓ Blood glucose regulation depends mainly on the hormones insulin and glucagon. Certain carbohydrate foods produce a greater rise and fall in blood glucose than others do. Most people have no problem regulating their blood glucose when they consume regular mixed meals.

✓ The liver converts extra energy compounds into fat, a more permanent and unlimited energy storage compound than glycogen and one that can be stored in almost unlimited quantities.

✓ Diabetes is an example of the body's abnormal handling of glucose. Inadequate or ineffective insulin leaves blood glucose high and cells undersupplied with glucose energy. This causes blood vessel and tissue damage. Weight control and exercise may be effective in preventing the predominant form of diabetes (type 2) and the illnesses that accompany it. A person diagnosed with diabetes must establish patterns of eating, exercise, and medication to control blood glucose.

✓ Postprandial hypoglycemia is a rare medical condition in which blood glucose falls too low. It can be a warning of organ damage or disease. Many people believe they experience symptoms of hypoglycemia, but their symptoms normally do not accompany below-normal blood glucose.

SUMMING UP

Carbohydrates are the first link in the food chain and are obtained almost exclusively from

(1) _____. Through (2) _____, plants combine carbon dioxide,

water, and the sun's energy to form (3) _____, from which the human body can

obtain energy. Carbohydrates are made of carbon, hydrogen, and (4) _____. Six sugar

molecules are important in nutrition, including three (5) _____ and three

disaccharides. The monosaccharides include glucose, galactose, and (6) _____; the

disaccharides include (7) _____, maltose, and (8) _____.

Glucose may be strung together in long strands to form (9) _____,

which include starch, glycogen, and most of the (10) _____. The best known

fibers are (11) _____, hemicellulose, and (12) _____.

Glucose from carbohydrate is the preferred (13) _____ for most body

functions; nerve cells, including those of the (14) _____ depend almost

exclusively on glucose for their energy. Government agencies in many countries urge their

citizens to consume foods that contain abundant (15) _____ carbohydrates

while the *World Health Organization* recommends (16) _____ percent of total

calories from complex carbohydrates.

Many different forms of fiber exist, each with their specific effects on health. The *World*

Health Organization recommends a daily intake of (17) _____ grams of dietary

fiber. Fiber needs are best met by eating (18) _____ foods;

The Carbohydrates: Sugar, Starch, Glycogen, and Fiber

(19) _____fiber in large doses can be harmful.

Glucose is the basic carbohydrate unit that each (20) _____ of the body

uses for energy. If the blood delivers more glucose than the cells need, the liver and

(21) _____ take up the surplus and build the polysaccharide (22) _____.

Without sufficient carbohydrate, the body turns to (23) _____ to make glucose.

Also, without sufficient carbohydrate, the body cannot use its (24) _____ in the

normal way.

Some people have physical conditions which cause abnormal handling of carbohydrates.

These conditions include (25) _____ intolerance, hypoglycemia, and

(26) _____. The predominant type of diabetes is (27) _____,

characterized by (28) _____ resistance of the body's cells. In contrast, the person

with type 1 diabetes secretes no (29)_____. The effects of diabetes can be severe

because the disease causes destruction or blockage of (30) _____ that feed the

body organs, and tissues die from lack of nourishment.

The term (31) _____ refers to abnormally low blood glucose. The two

types of hypoglycemia include postprandial and (32) _____. People who

experience the symptoms of hypoglycemia may benefit from eating regularly timed, balanced

(33) _____-containing meals and avoiding (34) _____beverages.

CHAPTER GLOSSARY

Matching Exercise 1:

_____ 1. monosaccharides

_____ 2. maltose

_____ 3. chelating agents

_____ 4. hemorrhoids

_____ 5. starch

_____ 6. appendicitis

_____ 7. polysaccharides

_____ 8. glucose

_____ 9. soluble fibers

_____ 10. diverticulosis

_____ 11. glycogen

_____ 12. fibers

_____ 13. sucrose

_____ 14. granules

_____ 15. insoluble fibers

a. compounds composed of long strands of glucose units linked together

b. molecules that surround other molecules and are therefore useful in either preventing or promoting movement of substances from place to place

c. a disaccharide composed of glucose and fructose

d. food components that readily dissolve in water and often impart gummy or gel-like characteristics to foods

e. a disaccharide composed of two glucose units

f. the tough, fibrous structures of fruits, vegetables, and grains; indigestible food components that do not dissolve in water

g. a plant polysaccharide composed of glucose; highly digestible by human beings

h. a polysaccharide composed of glucose, made and stored by liver and muscle tissues of human beings and animals as a storage form of glucose

i. packages of starch molecules; various plant species make granules of varying shapes

j. inflammation and/or infection of the appendix, a sac protruding from the intestine

k. a single sugar used in both plant and animal tissues for energy

l. outpocketing or ballooning out of areas of the intestinal wall, caused by weakening of the muscle layers that encase the intestine

m. the indigestible polysaccharides in food, comprised mostly of cellulose, hemicellulose, and pectin

n. swollen, hardened (varicose) veins in the rectum, usually caused by the pressure resulting from constipation

o. single sugar units

Matching Exercise 2:

_____ 1. glucagon

_____ 2. diabetes

_____ 3. type 1 diabetes

_____ 4. simple carbohydrates

_____ 5. postprandial hypoglycemia

_____ 6. complex carbohydrates

_____ 7. chlorophyll

_____ 8. hypoglycemia

_____ 9. fasting hypoglycemia

_____ 10. lactose intolerance

_____ 11. resistin

_____ 12. photosynthesis

_____ 13. glycemic effect

_____ 14. protein-sparing action

a. a disease characterized by elevated blood glucose and inadequate or ineffective insulin, which renders a person unable to regulate blood glucose normally

b. the green pigment of plants that captures energy from sunlight for use in photosynthesis

c. a hormone made and released by fat cells under conditions of obesity and thought to increase tissue resistance to the effects of insulin

d. the extent to which a food raises the blood glucose concentration and elicits an insulin response as compared with pure glucose

e. sugars, including both single sugar units and linked pairs of sugar units

f. hypoglycemia that occurs after 8 to 14 hours of fasting

g. the process by which green plants make carbohydrates from carbon dioxide and water using the green pigment chlorophyll to capture the sun's energy

h. a hormone secreted by the pancreas that stimulates the liver to release glucose into the blood when blood glucose concentration dips

i. long chains of sugar units arranged to form starch or fiber; also called *polysaccharides*

j. a blood glucose concentration below normal, a symptom that may indicate any of several diseases, including impending diabetes

k. the type of diabetes in which the person produces no or very little insulin

l. inability to digest lactose due to a lack of the enzyme lactase

m. a drop in blood glucose that follows a meal and is accompanied by symptoms of the stress response

n. the action of carbohydrate and fat in providing energy that allows protein to be used for purposes it alone can serve

Matching Exercise 3:

_____ 1. constipation

_____ 2. disaccharides

_____ 3. galactose

_____ 4. lactase

_____ 5. fructose

_____ 6. roughage

_____ 7. sugars

_____ 8. carbohydrates

_____ 9. lactose

_____ 10. glycemic index

_____ 11. type 2 diabetes

_____ 12. insulin

_____ 13. ketone bodies

_____ 14. ketosis

_____ 15. resistant starch

a. the rough parts of food; an imprecise term that has largely been replaced by the term *fiber*

b. a disaccharide composed of glucose and galactose; sometimes known as milk sugar

c. pairs of single sugars linked together

d. a monosaccharide; sometimes known as fruit sugar

e. monosaccharide; part of the disaccharide lactose

f. hardness and dryness of bowel movements; associated with discomfort in passing them from the body

g. an undesirable high concentration of ketone bodies, such as acetone, in the blood or urine

h. acidic, fat-related compounds that can arise from the incomplete breakdown of fat when carbohydrate is not available

i. hormone secreted by the pancreas in response to a high blood glucose concentration

j. the intestinal enzyme that splits the disaccharide lactose to monosaccharides during digestion

k. the type of diabetes in which the person makes plenty of insulin but the body cells resist insulin's action

l. simple carbohydrates, that is, molecules of either single sugar units or pairs of those sugar units bonded together

m. a ranked measure of the glycemic effect of foods

n. compounds composed of single or multiple sugars

o. the fraction of starch in a food that is digested slowly, or not at all, by human enzymes

EXERCISES

Answer these chapter study questions:

1. From a nutrition perspective, how do fruits differ from concentrated sweets?

2.   How does fiber help maintain a healthy body weight?

3.   Describe how the body adjusts after a meal when the blood glucose level rises.

4.   Why are fasting and low carbohydrate diets dangerous?

5.   Why can some people with lactose intolerance consume and tolerate yogurt or
      aged cheese?

Complete these short answer questions:

1. The only animal-derived food that contains significant amounts of carbohydrate is _____.

2. Carbohydrates are made of:

   a.
   b.
   c.

3. The monosaccharides include:

   a.
   b.
   c.

4. The disaccharides include:

   a.
   b.
   c.

5. Complex carbohydrates include:

   a.
   b.
   c.

6. The fibers of a plant contribute the supporting structures of its:

   a.
   b.
   c.

7. The best known of the fibers include:

   a.
   b.
   c.

8. Groups of individuals who are especially vulnerable to the adverse effects of excess fiber include:

   a.
   b.
   c.

9. A balanced diet that is high in _____ carbohydrate helps control body weight and maintain lean tissue.

10. An average-size person needs around _____ grams of carbohydrate per day to insure complete sparing of body protein and avoidance of ketosis.

Solve these problems:

1. Estimate the grams of dietary fiber and carbohydrate supplied by the following menu:

Breakfast	Fiber (grams)	Carbohydrate (grams)
1 cup skim milk	_____	_____
1 slice whole wheat toast	_____	_____
1 oz. cheddar cheese	_____	_____
1 medium orange	_____	_____

Lunch		
Salad with:		
2 cups raw lettuce	_____	_____
1 medium tomato	_____	_____
2 tbsp. oil and vinegar dressing	_____	_____
1 medium apple	_____	_____

Dinner		
3 oz. chicken breast	_____	_____
1/2 cup broccoli	_____	_____
1 medium baked potato with skin	_____	_____
1 slice rye bread	_____	_____
1 cup plain yogurt with	_____	_____
1/2 cup blackberries	_____	_____

TOTAL:	_____	_____

2. Use the ingredient label below to respond to the questions which follow.

> INGREDIENTS: *Bleached flour, sugar, partially hydrogenated vegetable shortening, dextrose, water, corn syrup, carob, whey blend, cornstarch, salt, sodium bicarbonate, lecithin, artificial flavoring and artificial colors.*

   a. List all of the sugars which appear in the above product.

   b. Would you consider this product to be high or low in sugar content? Why?

Solve these controversy questions:

1. What is primarily responsible for the steady, upward trend in U.S. sugar consumption?

2. Why does fat and total calorie intake usually rise when sugar intake increases?

3. How would you respond to someone who makes the statement that sugary foods cause children to become hyperactive and unruly?

4. If a person consumes 3,000 calories a day, how many calories from sugars could he/she consume to be in compliance with the World Health Organization's recommendations?

5.   Why is isomalt less likely than other sugar alcohols to cause diarrhea?

STUDY AIDS

1.   Identify whether the following health effects are characteristic of insoluble or soluble fiber by placing an X in those spaces answered with a yes response.

	Insoluble	Soluble
a. slows transit of food through the upper digestive tract	_____	_____
b. regular bowel movements	_____	_____
c. slows glucose absorption	_____	_____
d. lowers blood cholesterol	_____	_____

2.   Use the following tables in your textbook as study aids: Table 4-2 on page 107; Table 4-7 on page 118.

SAMPLE TEST ITEMS

Comprehension Level Items:

1.   Carbohydrate-rich foods are obtained almost exclusively from animals.

a.   true
b.   false

2.   Carbohydrates are made of the following:

a.   oxygen, nitrogen, and carbon
b.   nitrogen, hydrogen, and carbon
c.   hydrogen, carbon, and oxygen
d.   carbon dioxide, hydrogen, and oxygen

3. Fructose occurs in all of the following *except*:

   a. honey
   b. table sugar
   c. fruit
   d. milk

4. Maltose consists of:

   a. glucose and galactose
   b. galactose and fructose
   c. two glucose units
   d. lactose and glucose

5. Which of the following does *not* occur free in nature?

   a. fructose
   b. galactose
   c. sucrose
   d. glucose

6. Complex carbohydrates are called:

   a. natural sugars
   b. monosaccharides
   c. polysaccharides
   d. complex sugars

7. The storage form of glucose found in plants is called:

   a. starch
   b. cholorphyll
   c. fiber
   d. glycogen

8. Common uses of pectin include:

   a. to thicken jelly
   b. to keep salad dressing from separating
   c. to make milk more digestible
   d. a and b
   e. a and c

The Carbohydrates: Sugar, Starch, Glycogen, and Fiber

For questions 9–11, match the terms on the right with their definitions on the left.

9. _____ food components that readily dissolve in water and often impart gummy or gel-like characteristics to foods

10. _____ the indigestible polysaccharides in food

11. _____ the rough parts of food

a. fibers

b. residue

c. roughage

d. insoluble fibers

e. soluble fibers

12. The human brain depends almost exclusively on _____ for its energy.

   a. fat
   b. carbohydrate
   c. alcohol
   d. protein

13. Fiber promotes maintenance of proper weight through all of the following effects *except:*

   a. absorbing water and creating a feeling of fullness
   b. donating few calories
   c. speeding up movement of food through the upper digestive tract
   d. displacing calorie-dense concentrated fats and sweets from the diet

14. Which of the following parts of a wheat kernel is rich in both nutrients and fiber?

   a. endosperm
   b. germ
   c. husk
   d. bran

15. The body's form of stored glucose is called:

   a. glycogen
   b. starch
   c. glucagon
   d. ketones

16. Which of the following would you choose to lower your blood cholesterol level?

   a. purified fiber
   b. wheat bran
   c. brown rice
   d. oat bran

17. Which of the following foods would be most easily digested based on its starch content?

   a. corn
   b. lima beans
   c. white bread
   d. potato

18. On drinking milk, a person with lactose intolerance is likely to experience:

    a. vomiting
    b. diarrhea
    c. excessive gas
    d. a and b
    e. b and c

19. Possible effects of diabetes include:

    a. disease of the feet and legs
    b. cataracts in the eye
    c. cancer of the pancreas
    d. a and b
    e. b and c

20. Carbohydrate-containing foods appear in all of the following food groups *except:*

    a. milk, cheese and yogurt
    b. vegetables
    c. bread, cereal, rice and pasta
    d. fats and oils

21. A typical serving of fruit contributes about _____ grams of carbohydrate.

    a. 5
    b. 12
    c. 15
    d. 18

22. Honey is more healthy than white sugar.

    a. true
    b. false

Application Level Items:

23. Someone makes the statement that eating fruit is the same as eating a candy bar. Your response would be:

    a. fruits differ from candy bars in nutrient density
    b. the sugars of fruits are diluted in large volumes of water
    c. candy bars are packaged in fiber
    d. a and b
    e. b and c

24. Which of the following would you recommend as a calcium source for someone with lactose intolerance?

    a. milk
    b. yogurt with added milk solids
    c. aged cheese
    d. a and b
    e. b and c

25. Why would you recommend that someone *not* add purified fiber to the diet?

    a. it might displace nutrients from the diet
    b. it might easily be taken to the extreme
    c. it is very expensive and adversely affects the taste of foods
    d. a and b
    e. b and c

26. Whole wheat bread is superior to white bread because of this nutrient:

    a. iron
    b. riboflavin
    c. chromium
    d. niacin

27. What argument(s) would you use against following a low-carbohydrate diet?

    a. the body uses protein to make energy
    b. the body uses up its fat as an energy source
    c. the body cannot use its fat in the normal way
    d. a and b
    e. a and c

28. How many grams of carbohydrate and calories from carbohydrate are contained in the following meal: **1 cup skim milk; 3 oz. sirloin steak;1/2 cup rice; 1/2 cup winter squash; 1 slice whole wheat bread; 1 small apple?**

    a. 52 grams CHO; 208 calories
    b. 58 grams CHO; 232 calories
    c. 62 grams CHO; 248 calories
    d. 72 grams CHO; 288 calories

ANSWERS

SUMMING UP

(1) plants; (2) photosynthesis; (3) glucose; (4) oxygen; (5) monosaccharides; (6) fructose; (7) sucrose; (8) lactose; (9) polysaccharides; (10) fibers; (11) cellulose; (12) pectin; (13) fuel; (14) brain; (15) complex; (16) 50-75; (17) 27-40; (18) unprocessed; (19) purified; (20) cell; (21) muscles; (22) glycogen; (23) protein; (24) fat; (25) lactose; (26) diabetes; (27) type 2; (28) insulin; (29) insulin; (30) capillaries; (31) hypoglycemia; (32) fasting; (33) protein; (34) alcoholic

CHAPTER GLOSSARY

Matching Exercise 1: (1) o; (2) e; (3) b; (4) n; (5) g; (6) j; (7) a; (8) k; (9) d; (10) l; (11) h; (12) m; (13) c; (14) i; (15) f
Matching Exercise 2: (1) h; (2) a; (3) k; (4) e; (5) m; (6) i; (7) b; (8) j; (9) f; (10) l; (11) c; (12) g; (13) d; (14) n
Matching Exercise 3: (1) f; *(2)* c; (3) e; (4) j; (5) d; (6) a; (7) l; (8) n; (9) b; (10) m; (11) k; (12) i; (13) h; (14) g; (15) o

EXERCISES

Chapter Study Questions:

1. The sugars in fruits are diluted in large volumes of water, packaged with fiber, and are mixed with many vitamins and minerals needed by the body. Concentrated sweets are much less nutrient-dense and may also be high in fat.

2. Because high fiber foods absorb water, swell and create a feeling of fullness; in addition, they donate few calories and displace calorie-dense concentrated fats and sweets from the diet. Some fibers also slow movement of food through the upper digestive tract so that you feel fuller for a longer period of time.

3. The pancreas detects the excess glucose and releases the hormone insulin, which signals the body's tissues to take up surplus glucose. The body siphons off the excess into the liver, to be converted to glycogen or fat and into the muscle, to be converted to glycogen.

4. When there is a severe carbohydrate deficit, the body turns to protein to make glucose, thus diverting protein from its vitally important functions such as maintaining the body's immune defenses. Secondly, the body cannot use its fat in the normal way without sufficient carbohydrate and goes into ketosis, which disturbs the body's normal acid-base balance.

5. Because the bacteria or mold that helps create yogurt and aged cheese digest lactose as they convert milk to the fermented product.

Short Answer Questions:

1. milk

2. (a) carbon; (b) hydrogen; (c) oxygen

3. (a) glucose; (b) galactose; (c) fructose

4. (a) sucrose; (b) maltose; (c) lactose

5. (a) starch, (b) fiber; (c) glycogen

6. (a) leaves; (b) stems; (c) seeds

7. (a) cellulose; (b) hemicellulose; (c) pectin

8. (a) malnourished; (b) elderly; (c) children who consume no animal products

9. complex

10. 100

Problem-Solving:

1.

Breakfast	Fiber (grams)	Carbohydrate (grams)
1 cup skim milk		12
1 slice whole wheat toast	2	15
1oz. cheddar cheese		
1 medium orange	3	15

Lunch		
Salad with:		
2 cups raw lettuce	2	10
1 medium tomato	1	5
2 tbsp. oil and vinegar		
dressing		
1 medium apple	3	15

Dinner		
3 oz. chicken breast		
1/2 cup broccoli	2	5
1 medium baked potato with skin	5	15
1 slice rye bread	2	15
1 cup plain yogurt with		12
1/2 cup blackberries	4	15
TOTAL:	**24**	**134**

2. (a) sugar; dextrose; corn syrup; (b) high; because it contains three different sugars which appear as the second, fourth, and sixth ingredients on the label

Controversy Questions:

1. A dramatic increase in the purchase of commercially prepared foods and beverages to which sugars have been added.

2. Because sweet treats often contain abundant fat and calories

3. Studies have overwhelmingly failed to demonstrate any consistent effects of sucrose on behavior in either normal or hyperactive children.

4. 300 calories from sugar

5. Because its larger chemical structure attracts less water into the colon

STUDY AIDS

		Insoluble	Soluble
1.	a. slows transit of food through the upper digestive tract	_____	X
	b. regular bowel movements	X	_____
	c. slows glucose absorption	_____	X
	d. lowers blood cholesterol	_____	X

SAMPLE TEST ITEMS

1.	b (p. 100)	10.	a (p. 103)	19.	d (p. 119)
2.	c (p. 100)	11.	c (p. 103)	20.	d (p. 121)
3.	d (p. 101)	12.	b (p. 104)	21.	c (p. 121)
4.	c (p. 101)	13.	c (p. 105)	22.	b (p. 123-124)
5.	b (p. 101)	14.	d (p. 108)	23.	d (p. 101)
6.	c (p. 100)	15.	a (p. 115)	24.	c (p. 113)
7.	a (p. 102)	16.	d (p. 106)	25.	d (p. 107)
8.	d (p. 103)	17.	c (p. 111)	26.	c (p. 109)
9.	e (p. 103)	18.	e (p. 113)	27.	e (p. 114)
				28.	d (p 121)

CHAPTER 5

The Lipids: Fats, Oils, Phospholipids, and Sterols

CHAPTER OBJECTIVES

After completing this chapter, you should be able to:

1. Explain the way lipids are useful, both in foods and in the body.

2. Describe the structure of a triglyceride noting the differences between saturated and unsaturated fats.

3. Summarize the processes of lipid digestion, absorption, transport, and utilization in the body, including the significance of the lipoproteins.

4. Explain why manufacturers frequently hydrogenate fats and the possible health implications of consuming the trans-fatty acids formed during hydrogenation.

5. List the arguments for and against the growing use of the fat replacers.

6. Plan a diet containing fat in the right kinds and in the recommended amounts to provide optimal health and pleasure in eating.

7. Compare the Mediterranean Diet Pyramid with the USDA Food Guide Pyramid (Controversy 5).

KEY CONCEPTS

✓   Lipids not only serve as energy reserves but also cushion the vital organs, protect the body from temperature extremes, carry the fat-soluble nutrients, serve as raw materials, and provide the major component of cell membranes.

✓   Lipids provide more energy per gram than carbohydrate and protein, enhance food's aroma and flavor, and contribute to satiety, or a feeling of fullness, after a meal.

✓   The body combines three fatty acids with one glycerol to make a triglyceride, its storage form of fat. Fatty acids in food influence the composition of fats in the body.

✓   Fatty acids are energy-rich carbon chains that can be saturated (filled with hydrogens) or monounsaturated (with one point of unsaturation) or polyunsaturated (with more than one point of unsaturation). The degree of saturation of the fatty acids in a fat determines the fat's softness or hardness.

✓   Phospholipids, including lecithin, play key roles in cell membranes; sterols play roles as part of bile, vitamin D, the sex hormones, and other important compounds.

✓   In the stomach, fats separate from other food components. In the small intestine, bile emulsifies the fats, enzymes digest them, and the intestinal cells absorb them. Large lipids must be incorporated into chylomicrons for transport in the blood.

✓   Blood and other body fluids are watery, so fats need special transport vehicles -the lipoproteins- to carry them around the body in these fluids. The chief lipoproteins are chylomicrons, VLDL, LDL, and HDL.

✓   When low on fuel, the body draws on its stored fat for energy. Glucose is necessary for the complete breakdown of fat; without carbohydrate, ketosis occurs.

✓   The major dietary factor that raises blood cholesterol is the saturated fat intake, not the intake of cholesterol in foods. Elevated blood cholesterol is a risk factor for cardiovascular disease. Trimming fat from food trims calories and, often, saturated fat as well.

✓   Dietary measures to lower LDL in the blood involve reducing saturated fat and substituting monounsaturated and polyunsaturated fats for saturated fat. A few people must also reduce cholesterol intake. Cholesterol-containing foods are nutritious and are best used in moderation by most people.

✓   Two polyunsaturated fatty acids, linoleic acid (an omega-6 acid) and linolenic acid (an omega-3 acid), are essential nutrients used to make substances that perform many functions. The omega-6 family includes linoleic acid; seed oils are rich sources. The omega-3 family includes linolenic acid, EPA, and DHA. Fish oils are rich sources of EPA and DHA. Fish oil supplements are not recommended.

✓   Vegetable oils become more saturated when they are hydrogenated. Hydrogenated fats resist rancidity better, are firmer textured, and have a higher smoking point than unsaturated oil; but they also lose the health benefits of unsaturated oils.

✓   The process of hydrogenation creates trans-fatty acids. Trans-fatty acids act somewhat like saturated fats in the body.

✓ Fats added to foods during preparation or at the table are a major source of fat in the diet.

✓ Meats account for a large proportion of the hidden fat in many people's diets. Most people consume meat in larger servings than those recommended.

✓ The choice between whole and fat-free milk products can make a large difference to the fat content of a diet.

✓ Fat in breads and cereals can be well hidden. Consumers must learn which foods of this group contain fats.

SUMMING UP

Lipid is the general term for a family of organic compounds insoluble in (1) _____

and about 95 percent of the lipids in foods and in the human body are (2) _____.

Other classes of the lipid family include the phospholipids and the (3) _____.

     Although too much fat in the diet has the potential to be (4) _____,

lipids serve many valuable functions in the body. Fat is the body's chief storage form for

(5) _____ from food eaten in excess of need. In addition, fat surrounds and

cushions all the body's vital (6) _____ and insulates the body from extremes in

(7) _____. Some essential nutrients, such as the essential (8) _____ and

the fat-soluble vitamins A, D, E, and (9) _____, are found primarily in foods that

contain fat.

     Fatty acids are the major constituent of (10) _____, which are the chief

form of fat, and they differ from one another in two ways: in (11) _____ length

and in degree of (12) _____. The more unsaturated a fat, the more

(13) _____ it is at room temperature. Generally, vegetable and

(14) _____ oils are rich in polyunsaturates. However, two vegetable oils,

including coconut and (15) _____, are highly saturated.

     Within the body, many fats travel from place to place in blood as passengers in

(16) _____. The more protein in the lipoprotein molecule, the higher the

(17) _____. Two types of lipoproteins of concern to health care providers

include (18) _____ and (19) _____. Elevated HDL

concentrations are associated with a (20) _____ risk of heart attack. High blood

(21) _____ is an indicator of risk for CVD and the main dietary factor

associated with elevated blood cholesterol is a high (22) _____ intake.

Two fatty acids, including linoleic and (23) _____, must be supplied by

the diet and are, therefore, (24) _____ fatty acids. Points of unsaturation in fatty

acids are vulnerable to attack by (25) _____ and when the unsaturated points are

oxidized, the oils become (26) _____. Cooking oils should be stored in tightly

covered containers that exclude (27) _____. One way to prevent spoilage of

unsaturated fats and also to make them harder is to change their fatty acids chemically by

(28) _____. The process of hydrogenation creates (29) _____,

which act somewhat like saturated fats in the body.

Fats added to foods during (30) _____ or at the table are a major

source of fat in the diet. Fats may be (31) _____ on foods, such as the fat

trimmed from a steak, or they may be invisible, such as the fat in biscuits or olives.

CHAPTER GLOSSARY

Matching Exercise 1:

_____ 1. phospholipids	a. lipids that are solid at room temperature (70°F or 25°C)
_____ 2. fats	b. an emulsifier made by the liver from cholesterol and stored in the gallbladder
_____ 3. lipid	c. one of the three main classes of dietary lipids and the chief form of fat in foods
_____ 4. oils	d. a fatty acid containing one point of unsaturation
_____ 5. cholesterol	e. a substance that mixes with both fat and water and permanently disperses the fat in the water, forming an emulsion
_____ 6. emulsifier	f. one of the three main classes of dietary lipids; these lipids are similar to triglycerides, but each has a phosphorus containing acid in place of one of the fatty acids
_____ 7. sterols	g. lipids that are liquid at room temperature (70°F or 25°C)
_____ 8. polyunsaturated fatty acid	h. a fatty acid carrying the maximum possible number of hydrogen atoms
_____ 9. bile	i. products of the digestion of lipids
_____ 10. saturated fatty acid	j. a phospholipid manufactured by the liver and also found in many foods; a major constituent of cell membranes
_____ 11. monounsaturated fatty acid	k. a family of compounds soluble in organic solvents but not in water
_____ 12. lecithin	l. a fatty acid that lacks some hydrogen atoms and has one or more points of unsaturation
_____ 13. unsaturated fatty acid	m. a fatty acid with two or more points of unsaturation
_____ 14. monoglycerides	n. an organic compound, three carbons long, of interest here because it serves as the backbone for triglycerides
_____ 15. glycerol	o. one of the three main classes of dietary lipids, with a structure similar to that of cholesterol
_____ 16. triglycerides	p. a member of the group of lipids known as sterols; a soft waxy substance made in the body for a variety of purposes and also found in animal derived foods
_____ 17. cardiovascular disease	q. triglycerides in which most of the fatty acids are saturated
_____ 18. saturated fats	r. disease of the heart and blood vessels

Matching Exercise 2:

_____ 1. trans-fatty acids

_____ 2. smoking point

_____ 3. dietary antioxidants

_____ 4. essential fatty acids

_____ 5. fatty acids

_____ 6. HDL

_____ 7. lipoproteins

_____ 8. oxidation

_____ 9. satiety

_____ 10. artificial fats

_____ 11. omega-6 fatty acid

_____ 12. hydrogenation

_____ 13. omega-3 fatty acid

_____ 14. chylomicrons

_____ 15. LDL

_____ 16. fat replacer

_____ 17. stanol esters

a. the feeling of fullness or satisfaction that people experience after meals

b. the temperature at which fat gives off an acrid blue gas

c. clusters formed when lipids from a meal are combined with carrier proteins in the intestinal lining

d. organic acids composed of carbon chains of various lengths

e. an ingredient that replaces some or all of the functions of fat and may or may not provide energy

f. fatty acids that the body needs but cannot make in amounts sufficient to meet physiological needs

g. clusters of lipids associated with protein, which serve as transport vehicles for lipids in blood and lymph

h. the process of adding hydrogen to unsaturated fatty acids to make fat more solid and resistant to the chemical change of oxidation

i. fatty acids with unusual shapes that can arise when polyunsaturated oils are hydrogenated

j. zero-energy fat replacers that are chemically synthesized to mimic the sensory and cooking qualities of naturally occurring fats, but are totally or partially resistant to digestion

k. lipoproteins containing a large proportion of cholesterol that transport lipids from the liver to other tissues such as muscle and fat

l. interaction of a compound with oxygen

m. a polyunsaturated fatty acid with its endmost double bond three carbons from the end of its carbon chain

n. lipoproteins containing a large proportion of protein that return cholesterol from storage places to the liver for dismantling and disposal

o. substances in food that significantly decrease the damaging effects of reactive compounds, such as reactive forms of oxygen and nitrogen on tissue functioning

p. a polyunsaturated fatty acid with its endmost double bond six carbons from the end of the carbon chain

q. plant-derived compounds belonging to the sterol family of lipids that have been shown experimentally to reduce blood cholesterol when consumed in place of other fats in a low-fat diet

EXERCISES

Answer these chapter study questions:

1. Why is fat, rather than carbohydrate, the body's major form of stored energy?

2. Why are oils vulnerable to rancidity and how can rancidity be retarded?

3. Why do vegetable oils make up most of the added fat in the U.S. diet?

4. Identify the best way to raise HDL and dietary measures to decrease LDL.

5. What is the ideal ratio of intake of omega-3 to omega-6 fatty acids and what is the best way to obtain the right balance?

Complete these short answer questions:

1. The three major classes of lipids include:

    a.
    b.
    c.

2. Triglycerides are made up of three _____ units and _____ glycerol unit.

3. Identify three useful functions of fats in foods.

    a.
    b.
    c.

4. Fatty acids may differ from one another in two ways:

    a.
    b.

5. The two fatty acids essential for human beings include:

    a.
    b.

6. Identify two vegetable oils which are saturated fats:

    a.
    b.

7. Three advantages of hydrogenated oils are:

    a.
    b.
    c.

The Lipids: Fats, Oils, Phospholipids, and Sterols

8. The two major types of lipoproteins of concern to health care professionals include:

    a.
    b.

9. The main dietary factor associated with elevated blood cholesterol is a high _____ intake.

10. Two groups in the *Food Guide Pyramid* that always contain fat include:

    a.
    b.

Solve these problems:

1. Using the exchange lists, calculate the number of grams of fat in the following breakfast menu:

Item	_Grams of Fat_
2 strips of crisp bacon	_____
2 eggs scrambled with 2 teaspoons margarine	_____
1/2 cup oatmeal	_____
1 slice of toast with 1 teaspoon margarine	_____
1 cup 2% milk	_____
TOTAL:	_____

2. Circle all of the words in the label below which alert you to the fat content of the product.

> *INGREDIENTS: Chicken stock, chicken, wheat flour, corn starch, cream, vegetable oil, salt, chicken fat, water, margarine, monosodium glutamate, soy protein isolate, yeast extract and natural flavoring.*

3. Modify the following recipe for Beef Stroganoff by making substitutions for the high fat ingredients.

Traditional Recipe

1 pound ground beef
1/2 cup chopped onion
1 small clove garlic, minced
1 jar sliced mushrooms, drained
2 tablespoons butter
2 tablespoons all-purpose flour
8 ounce carton sour cream
1/4 cup chili sauce
1/2 teaspoon Worcestershire sauce
1 teaspoon salt
1/4 teaspoon pepper

Modifications:_____

_____

_____

Solve these controversy questions:

1. What is the primary evidence that supports the idea that the Mediterranean diet, rather than genetics, is the primary variable that confers disease risk or protection?

2. What are the eight attributes of the Mediterranean diet thought to be responsible for its health-promoting characteristics?

3. Why is a high intake of vegetables correlated with a low incidence of chronic diseases?

4. What scientific evidence supports the health benefits of consuming olive oil?

5. What is the most controversial suggestion of the Mediterranean Pyramid and why?

STUDY AIDS

Use the following table and figure in your textbook as study aids: Table 5-1 on page 140; Figure 5-5 on page 143.

SAMPLE TEST ITEMS

Comprehension Level Items:

1. Which of the following is ***not*** one of the three main classes of lipids?

   a. triglycerides
   b. lecithin
   c. phospholipids
   d. sterols

2. Lecithin is an example of a:

    a. phospholipid
    b. triglyceride
    c. sterol
    d. fatty acid

3. Which of the following is *not* a characteristic of fat in food or in the body?

    a. provides energy reserves
    b. protects the body from temperature extremes
    c. helps cushion vital body organs
    d. decreases the flavor of foods
    e. forms the major material of cell membranes

4. A saturated fatty acid is a fatty acid:

    a. possessing an "empty spot"
    b. having two or more points of unsaturation
    c. carrying the maximum possible number of hydrogen atoms
    d. a and b
    e. b and c

5. The essential fatty acids include:

    a. linoleic acid
    b. linolenic acid
    c. arachidonic acid
    d. a and b
    e. b and c

6. Which of the following helps prevent spoilage of oils containing unsaturated fatty acids?

    a. change them chemically by hydrogenation
    b. make them more unsaturated
    c. add an antioxidant
    d. a and b
    e. a and c

7. Of the following fats, which is the hardest?

    a. safflower oil
    b. chicken fat
    c. lard
    d. coconut oil

8. A person who eats a high-fat diet incurs a greater-than-average risk of developing:

    a. heart disease
    b. osteoporosis
    c. cancer
    d. a and b
    e. a and c

The Lipids: Fats, Oils, Phospholipids, and Sterols

9. Within the body, fats usually travel from place to place mixed with _____ particles.

    a. carbohydrate
    b. protein
    c. glycerol
    d. glycogen

10. Which of the following statements concerning cholesterol is *__not__* true?

    a. it is the major part of the plaques that narrow the arteries
    b. it is widespread in the body and necessary to its function
    c. it is an important sterol in the structure of brain and nerve cells
    d. it cannot be made by the body and must be consumed in the diet

11. The main dietary factor associated with elevated blood cholesterol levels is:

    a. high total fat intake
    b. monounsaturated fats
    c. dietary cholesterol
    d. high saturated fat intake

12. Which of the following foods are considered to be fat-free?

    a. fruits
    b. milk
    c. unprocessed vegetables
    d. a and b
    e. a and c

13. One teaspoon of oil or shortening donates _____ calories.

    a. 25
    b. 30
    c. 40
    d. 45

14. Which of the following is a true statement regarding olestra?

    a. it has not been approved by the FDA
    b. it passes through the digestive tract unabsorbed
    c. it has no side effects
    d. it has been proven safe for use with growing children

15. A blood lipid profile reveals much useful information regarding a person's risk of:

    a. diabetes
    b. cancer
    c. heart disease
    d. hypoglycemia

16. In most people, saturated fats raise blood cholesterol _____ dietary cholesterol.

    a. more than
    b. less than
    c. the same as
    d. much less than

17. Saturation refers to the number of _____ the fatty acid chain is holding.

    a. oxygens
    b. hydrogens
    c. glycerols
    d. nitrogens

18. Trans-fatty acids act somewhat like _____ fats in the body.

    a. saturated
    b. unsaturated
    c. monounsaturated
    d. polyunsaturated

19. Linolenic acid, EPA and DHA are examples of:

    a. omega-6 fatty acids
    b. linoleic acid
    c. polyunsaturated fatty acids
    d. omega-3 fatty acids

Application Level Items:

20. Someone asks you whether he should reduce dietary cholesterol in an effort to prevent cardiovascular disease. An appropriate response would be:

    a. cholesterol, in general, doesn't matter
    b. it doesn't matter as much as saturated fat intake
    c. dietary cholesterol makes a major contribution
    d. very few foods contain cholesterol anyway

21. You are trying to get a group of people to reduce their fat intake. You tell them that the most effective step they can take at home is to:

    a. replace butter with margarine
    b. eat fewer foods
    c. eliminate fats used as seasonings
    d. consume fewer snacks throughout the day

22. Research suggests that North Americans should consume more omega-3 fatty acids. In order to do this, you would consume more:

    a. beef
    b. safflower oil
    c. corn oil
    d. salmon

23. You are trying to convince a friend not to buy fish oil supplements. You would use all of the following as arguments *except*:

    a. concentrated supplements make it easy to overdose on toxic vitamins
    b. the supplements are very expensive
    c. overdoses may cause heart disease and cancer
    d. supplements may have toxic concentrations of pesticides

24. A person recently had a blood lipid profile with these values: total cholesterol 350 mg/dl; LDL 140 mg/dl; HDL 25 mg/dl. Would this person be considered at risk for heart disease?

    a. yes
    b. no

25. Which of the following would provide the least amount of trans-fatty acids?

    a. peanut butter
    b. blue cheese salad dressing
    c. liquid margarine
    d. potato chips

ANSWERS

SUMMING UP

(1) water; (2) triglycerides; (3) sterols; (4) harmful; (5) energy; (6) organs; (7) temperature; (8) fatty acids; (9) K; (10) triglycerides; (11) chain; (12) saturation; (13) liquid; (14) fish; (15) palm; (16) lipoproteins; (17) density; (18) LDL; (19) HDL; (20) low; (21) cholesterol; (22) saturated fat; (23) linolenic; (24) essential; (25) oxygen; (26) rancid; (27) air; (28) hydrogenation; (29) trans-fatty acids; (30) preparation; (31) visible

CHAPTER GLOSSARY

Matching Exercise 1: (1) f; (2) a; (3) k; (4) g; (5) p; (6) e; (7) o; (8) m; (9) b; (10) h; (11) d; (12) j; (13) l; (14) i; (15) n; (16) c ; (17) r; (18) q
Matching Exercise 2: (1) i; (2) b; (3) o; (4) f; (5) d; (6) n; (7) g; (8) l; (9) a; (10) j; (11) p; (12) h; (13) m; (14) c; (15) k; (16) e; (17) q

EXERCISES

Chapter Study Questions:

1. Glycogen, the stored form of carbohydrate, holds a great deal of water and is quite bulky. Therefore, the body cannot store enough glycogen to provide energy for very long. In contrast, fats pack tightly together without water and can store many more calories of energy in a small space.

2. Oils contain points of unsaturation in the fatty acids and these are vulnerable to attack by oxygen. When the unsaturated points are oxidized, the oils become rancid. To prevent rancidity, oils should be stored in tightly covered containers that exclude air and they should be placed in the refrigerator if stored for long periods of time.

3. Because fast food chains use them for frying, manufacturers add them to processed foods, and consumers tend to choose margarine over butter.

4. To raise HDL, people should exercise more; to decrease LDL, people should reduce saturated fat and substitute monounsaturated and polyunsaturated fats for saturated fat.

5. The ratio should be about 1 to 5; to obtain this balance, you should eat meals of fish 2-3 times a week, as well as small amounts of vegetable oils.

Short Answer Questions:

1. (a) triglycerides; (b) phospholipids; (c) sterols

2. fatty acid; one

3. (a) provide a concentrated energy source in foods; (b) enhance food's aroma and flavor; (c) contribute to satiety

4. (a) in chain length; (b) in degree of saturation

5. (a) linoleic; (b) linolenic

6. (a) coconut oil; (b) palm oil

7. (a) resist rancidity; (b) firm texture; (c) have a high smoking point

8. (a) LDL; (b) HDL

9. saturated fat

10. (a) fats; (b) meats

Problem-Solving:

1.

Item	Grams of Fat
2 strips of crisp bacon	10
2 eggs scrambled with 2 teaspoons margarine	20
1/2 cup oatmeal	0-1
1 slice of toast with 1 teaspoon margarine	5-6
1 cup 2% milk	5
TOTAL:	40

2. Chicken stock; chicken; cream; vegetable oil; chicken fat; margarine

3. Use round steak instead of ground beef; use reduced calorie margarine in the place of butter; use yogurt instead of sour cream.

Controversy Questions:

1. Because Mediterranean immigrants to the United States who adopt an American diet and lifestyle suffer heart disease and cancer at the same rates as native-born U.S. citizens

2. The diet is low in saturated fats, low in meats and meat products, high in legumes, high in grains, high in fruits, high in vegetables, moderate in milk and milk products, and moderate in alcohol.

3. Vegetables provide fiber, phytochemicals, antioxidants, and other nutrients and are also low in fat.

4. Olive oil is metabolized differently in the body and may conserve the beneficial blood lipid, HDL, while lowering levels of the riskier types of blood lipids; they also contain potent antioxidants and are resistant to oxidation which is a possible cause of heart disease

5. The most controversial suggestion is the advice to partake moderately of wine because it may invite development of alcoholism and an increase in alcohol-related traffic accidents.

SAMPLE TEST ITEMS

1. b (p. 138)
2. a (p. 138)
3. d (p. 138-140)
4. c (p. 141)
5. d (p. 152)
6. e (p. 155-156)
7. c (p. 141-142)
8. e (p. 148)
9. b (p. 145)
10. d (p. 144)
11. d (p. 148)
12. e (p. 157)
13. d (p. 157)
14. b (p. 158-160)
15. c (p. 148)
16. a (p. 148)
17. b (p. 141)
18. a (p. 156)
19. d (p. 154)
20. b (p. 148)
21. c (p. 150)
22. d (p. 154)
23. c (p. 153-154)
24. a (p. 151)
25. c (156-157)

CHAPTER 6

The Proteins and Amino Acids

CHAPTER OBJECTIVES

After completing this chapter, you should be able to:

1. Describe the structure of proteins and explain why adequate amounts of all the essential amino acids are required for protein synthesis.

2. Summarize the processes of protein digestion and absorption in the body.

3. Explain the roles of protein in the body.

4. Discuss the importance of protein quality and mutual supplementation.

5. Calculate your individual protein RDA and describe how nitrogen balance studies are used in determining the RDA for protein.

6. Describe the consequences of both protein deficiency and protein excess.

7. Compare the positive health aspects of a vegetarian diet with those of a diet that includes meat and describe ways each diet can include adequate nutrients. (Controversy 6)

KEY CONCEPTS

✓ Proteins are unique among the energy nutrients in that they possess nitrogen-containing amine groups and are composed of as many as 20 different amino acid units. Of the 20 amino acids, some are essential, and some are essential only in special circumstances.

✓ Amino acids link into long strands that coil and fold to make a wide variety of different proteins.

✓ Each type of protein has a distinctive sequence of amino acids and so has great specificity. Cells specialize in synthesizing only particular types of proteins.

✓ Proteins can be denatured by heat, acids, bases, alcohol, or the salts of heavy metals. Denaturation begins the process of digesting food protein and can also destroy body proteins.

✓ Digestion of protein involves denaturation by stomach acid, then enzymatic digestion in the stomach and small intestine to amino acids, dipeptides, and tripeptides.

✓ The cells of the small intestine complete digestion, absorb amino acids and some larger peptides, and release them into the bloodstream.

✓ The body needs amino acids to grow new cells and to replace worn-out ones.

✓ The body makes enzymes, hormones, and chemical messengers of the nervous system from its amino acids.

✓ Antibodies are formed from amino acids to defend against foreign proteins and other foreign substances within the body.

✓ Proteins help to regulate the body's electrolytes and fluids.

✓ Proteins buffer the blood against excess acidity or alkalinity.

✓ When the carbohydrate and fat consumed are insufficient to meet the body's energy need, food protein and body protein are sacrificed to supply energy. The nitrogen part is removed from each amino acid, and the resulting fragment is oxidized for energy.

✓ Amino acids can be metabolized to protein, nitrogen plus energy, glucose, or fat. They will be metabolized to protein only if sufficient energy is present from other sources. The diet should supply all essential amino acids and an adequate quantity of protein.

✓ The body's use of a protein depends in part on the user's health and on the protein's digestibility. To be used efficiently, protein should be accompanied by all the other nutrients.

✓ A protein's amino acid assortment greatly influences its usefulness to the body. Proteins lacking needed amino acids can be used only if those amino acids are present from other sources.

✓ The quality of a protein is measured by its amino acids, by its digestibility, or by how well it supports growth.

✓ Nitrogen balance compares nitrogen excreted from the body with nitrogen ingested in food. The amount of protein needed daily depends on size and stage of growth. The 1989 RDA for adults is 0.8 grams of protein per kilogram of body weight.

✓ Protein-deficiency symptoms are always observed when either protein or energy is deficient. Extreme food-energy deficiency is marasmus; extreme protein deficiency is kwashiorkor. The two diseases overlap most of the time, and together are called PEM.

✓ Health risks may follow the overconsumption of protein-rich foods.

SUMMING UP

Protein is a compound composed of carbon, hydrogen, oxygen, and (1)_____

atoms. Protein is made up of building blocks called (2) _____. About

(3) _____ amino acids, each with its different side chain, make up most of the

proteins of living tissue. The side chains make the amino acids differ in size,

(4)_____, and electrical charge.

      There are some amino acids that the healthy adult body makes too slowly or cannot make

at all and these are called the (5) _____ amino acids. In the first step of making a

protein, each amino acid is hooked to the next. A bond, called a (6) _____ bond,

is formed between the amine group end of one and the (7) _____ group end of

the next. The dramatically different (8) _____ of proteins enable them to

perform different tasks in the body. Among the most fascinating of the proteins are the

(9) _____, which act on other substances to change them chemically.

      Proteins can be denatured by heat, alcohol, (10) _____, bases, or the

salts of heavy metals. During digestion of proteins, an early step is denaturation by the

(11) _____. In the stomach, the (12) _____ helps to uncoil the

protein's strands so that the stomach enzymes can attack the peptide bonds. The stomach lining,

which is made partly of (13) _____, is protected by a coat of

(14)_____. Continual digestion, and finally absorption, of protein takes place in

the (15) _____.

The Proteins and Amino Acids

Protein serves many roles, including the support of (16) _____ and the maintenance of fluid and electrolyte and (17) _____ balance. If insufficient fat and (18) _____ foods are eaten, protein will be sacrificed to provide needed (19) _____. When amino acids are degraded for energy, their (20)_____ groups are stripped off and used elsewhere or incorporated by the liver into (21) _____ to be excreted in the urine.

Generally, amino acids from (22) _____ proteins are best absorbed. If an (23) _____ amino acid is missing from food, the cells begin to adjust their activities almost immediately. The (24) _____ is the most important method of evaluating the quality of food protein and is used by those establishing protein values on food labels. However, the (25) _____ is used for measuring the protein quality of infant formulas and baby foods. On the PDCAAS scale of 100 to 0, with 100 representing protein sources that are most readily (26)_____and most perfectly balanced, (27) _____ , ground beef, chicken products, fat-free milk and (28) _____ all score 100.

The RDA for protein depends on (29) _____ and it is higher for (30) _____ and pregnant and lactating women to cover needs for building new tissue. For healthy adults, the RDA for protein has been set at (31) _____ grams for each kilogram of body weight.

Two groups of foods in the *Food Guide Pyramid* contribute high-quality protein, including the (32) _____ group and the meat group. In addition, the vegetable and (33) _____ groups contribute smaller amounts of proteins. Protein-rich foods carry with them a characteristic array of vitamins and (34) _____, including vitamin B$_{12}$, and (35) _____.

CHAPTER GLOSSARY

Matching Exercise 1:

_____ 1. immunity

_____ 2. peptide bond

_____ 3. polypeptides

_____ 4. essential amino acids

_____ 5. bases

_____ 6. edema

_____ 7. dipeptides

_____ 8. hormones

_____ 9. enzymes

_____ 10. amino acids

_____ 11. acid-base balance

_____ 12. fluid and electrolyte balance

_____ 13. proteins

_____ 14. acids

_____ 15. hemoglobin

_____ 16. side chain

_____ 17. denaturation

_____ 18. antibodies

a. chemical messengers secreted by a number of body organs in response to conditions that require regulation

b. compounds composed of carbon, hydrogen, oxygen, and nitrogen and arranged as strands of amino acids

c. protein fragments of many (more than ten) amino acids bonded together

d. large proteins of the blood, produced by the immune system in response to invasion of the body by foreign substances (antigens)

e. specific disease resistance, derived from the immune system's memory of prior exposure to specific disease agents and its ability to mount a swift defense against them

f. building blocks of protein

g. the unique chemical structure attached to the backbone of each amino acid that differentiates one amino acid from another

h. swelling of body tissue caused by leakage of fluid from the blood vessels

i. distribution of fluid and dissolved particles among body compartments

j. amino acids that either cannot be synthesized at all by the body or cannot be synthesized in amounts sufficient to meet physiological need

k. the globular protein of red blood cells whose iron atoms carry oxygen around the body

l. a bond that connects one amino acid with another, forming a link in a protein chain

m. compounds that release hydrogens in a watery solution

n. protein catalysts

o. the change in a protein's shape brought about by heat, acids, bases, alcohol, salts of heavy metals, or other agents

p. equilibrium between acid and base concentrations in the body fluids

q. protein fragments that are two amino acids long

r. compounds that accept hydrogens from solutions

Matching Exercise 2:

_____ 1. PER

_____ 2. kwashiorkor

_____ 3. tofu

_____ 4. acidosis

_____ 5. marasmus

_____ 6. urea

_____ 7. buffers

_____ 8. alkalosis

_____ 9. textured vegetable protein

_____ 10. limiting amino acid

_____ 11. dysentery

_____ 12. legumes

_____ 13. mutual supplementation

_____ 14. PDCAAS

_____ 15. complementary proteins

_____ 16. amine group

a. the strategy of combining two incomplete protein sources so that the amino acids in one food make up for those lacking in the other food

b. the calorie-deficiency disease; starvation

c. the nitrogen-containing portion of an amino acid

d. a curd made from soybean that is rich in protein, often rich in calcium and variable in fat content

e. an infection of the digestive tract that causes diarrhea

f. blood alkalinity above normal

g. a disease related to protein malnutrition, with a set of recognizable symptoms, such as edema

h. plants of the bean, pea, and lentil family that have roots with nodules containing special bacteria

i. processed soybean protein used in products formulated to look and taste like meat, fish,or poultry

j. a measuring tool used to determine protein quality; reflects a protein's digestibility as well as the proportions of amino acids that it provides

k. blood acidity above normal, indicating excess acid

l. compounds that help keep a solution's acidity or alkalinity constant

m. an essential amino acid present in dietary protein in an insufficient amount, so that it limits the body's ability to build protein

n. two or more proteins whose amino acid assortments complement each other in such a way that the essential amino acids missing from one are supplied by the other

o. the principal nitrogen-excretion product of metabolism, generated mostly by removal of amine groups from unneeded amino acids or from amino acids being sacrificed to a need for energy

p. a measure of protein quality assessed by determining how well a given protein supports weight gain in growing rats;used to judge the quality of protein in infant formulas and baby foods

EXERCISES

Answer these chapter study questions:

1. Why is milk given as a first-aid remedy when someone swallows a heavy-metal poison?

2. Describe the conditions under which amino acids would be wasted (e.g. not used to build protein).

3. Describe the main difference between these two methods of evaluating the quality of food protein: PDCAAS and PER.

4. What are legumes and why are they especially protein-rich food sources?

5. Why is it nutritionally advantageous to cook an egg?

Complete these short answer questions:

1. Proteins contain the following types of atoms:

    a.
    b.
    c.
    d.

2. The nine essential amino acids for adults include:

    a.   f.
    b.   g.
    c.   h.
    d.   i.
    e.

3. Amino acids in the cell can be:

    a.
    b.
    c.
    d.
    e.
    f.

4. Protein can undergo denaturation by:

    a.
    b.
    c.
    d.
    e.

5. Examples of proteins that contain ample amounts of all the essential amino acids include:

    a.   e.
    b.   f.
    c.   g.
    d.

6. Ways of evaluating the quality of food protein include:

    a.
    b.

7. List the steps necessary to calculate a person's RDA for protein.

    a.
    b.
    c.

8. The food groups in the *Food Guide Pyramid* which contribute protein to the diet include:

    a.
    b.
    c.
    d.

9. Protein-rich foods are notoriously lacking in the nutrients _____ and _____.

10. Protein-rich foods are high in vitamin _____ and the mineral _____.

Solve these problems:

1. What is the RDA for protein for a 37 year old female who is 5'4" tall and weighs 110 pounds?

2. Calculate the number of grams of protein provided in the following menu, using the exchange system.

Menu Item	Grams of Protein
Breakfast	
1 cup skim milk	_____
1 boiled egg	_____
1 slice whole wheat toast	_____
Lunch	
3 oz. hamburger patty	_____
1 whole wheat bun	_____
tomato and lettuce (1 vegetable serving)	_____
2 tsp. mayonnaise	_____
Dinner	
3 oz. chicken breast	_____
1/2 cup green beans	_____
1 roll	_____
1 cup skim milk	_____
Total:	_____

Solve these controversy questions:

1. What are some of the different reasons why individuals are vegetarians?

2. What are six conditions that a vegetarian diet may offer protection against?

3. Other than food choices, how do vegetarians differ from non-vegetarians?

4. How does the diet of people with colon cancer differ from those without colon cancer?

5. Which nutrients require special attention for strict vegetarians?

STUDY AIDS

1. Complete the blanks in the following table to illustrate traditional complementary protein combinations.

    a. black beans   plus _____
    b. bread   plus _____
    c. tofu   plus _____

2. Rank the following food items according to their PDCAAS values by placing a one next to the item with the highest score, a two next to the item with the next highest score, etc…

    _____ soybean protein
    _____ wheat protein
    _____ egg white

3. Use the following table and figure in your textbook as study aids: Table 6-1 on page 188; Figure 6-12 on page 189.

SAMPLE TEST ITEMS

Comprehension Level Items:

1. A strand of amino acids that makes up a protein may contain _____ different kinds of amino acids.

    a. 5
    b. 10
    c. 15
    d. 20

2. Which of the following makes amino acids differ in size, shape, and electrical charge?

    a. the side chains
    b. the amine groups
    c. the acid groups
    d. a and b
    e. b and c

3. Which of the following is **not** considered to be an essential amino acid?

    a. threonine
    b. alanine
    c. lysine
    d. phenylalanine

4. The body does **not** make a specialized storage form of protein as it does for carbohydrate and fat.

    a. true
    b. false

5. Appropriate roles of protein in the body include all of the following **except**:

    a. to provide the body's needed energy
    b. for growth and development
    c. to maintain fluid and electrolyte balance
    d. for acid-base balance

6. When there is a surplus of amino acids and energy-yielding nutrients, the body:

    a. removes and excretes their amine groups
    b. uses them to build extra muscle tissue
    c. converts them to fat for storage
    d. a and b
    e. a and c

7. Athletes need slightly more protein than the RDA, but the increased need is well covered by a regular diet.

    a. true
    b. false

8. Which of the following methods of evaluating protein quality is used as a standard for the majority of food labeling?

    a. chemical score
    b. net protein utilization
    c. protein efficiency ratio
    d. protein digestibility-corrected amino acid score

9. Of the following foods, which contains amino acids that are best digested and absorbed?

    a. whole wheat bread
    b. chicken
    c. legumes
    d. broccoli

10. The calorie deficiency disease is known as:

    a. protein-energy malnutrition
    b. kwashiorkor
    c. protein-calorie malnutrition
    d. marasmus

11. Characteristics of children with marasmus include all of the following *except*:

    a. their digestive enzymes are in short supply
    b. they retain some of their stores of body fat
    c. all of their muscles are wasted
    d. their metabolism is slowed

12. Under normal circumstances, healthy adults are in:

    a. nitrogen equilibrium
    b. positive nitrogen balance
    c. negative nitrogen balance
    d. minus zero balance

13. Which of the following is in positive nitrogen balance?

    a. a growing child
    b. a person who rests in bed for a long time
    c. a pregnant woman
    d. a and b
    e. a and c

14. High-protein diets are associated with all of the following *except*:

    a. high fat foods
    b. increased risk of obesity
    c. improved kidney function
    d. increased risk of heart disease

15. U.S. protein recommendations set an upper limit for protein intake of no more than twice the 1989 RDA amount.

    a. true
    b. false

16. Which of the following is *not* characteristic of legumes?

    a. they have nodules on their roots containing bacteria that can fix nitrogen
    b. they capture nitrogen from the air and soil and use it to make amino acids
    c. they are used by farmers in rotation with other crops to fertilize fields
    d. their protein quality is inferior to that of other plant foods

17. Heavy use of soy products in place of meat may severely inhibit _____ absorption.

    a. zinc
    b. vitamin C
    c. iron
    d. vitamin B$_{12}$

18. Tofu is:

    a. low in calcium
    b. a curd made from soybeans
    c. a poor source of protein
    d. high in fiber

19. These food groups contribute an abundance of high-quality protein:

    a. meat, poultry, fish, dry beans, eggs and nuts
    b. bread, cereal, rice and pasta
    c. milk, yogurt and cheese
    d. a and b
    e. a and c

Application Level Items:

20. Your best friend is a body builder who puts raw eggs in a milkshake to increase his protein intake. What argument would you use against this practice?

    a. raw egg proteins bind the B vitamin biotin
    b. raw egg proteins speed up protein digestion
    c. raw egg proteins bind the mineral iron
    d. a and b
    e. a and c

21. A person who centers his diet around protein is likely to receive an inadequate intake of:

    a. vitamin B$_{12}$
    b. fat
    c. folate
    d. iron

22. Valuable, expensive protein-rich foods can contribute to obesity when:

    a. there is a surplus of amino acids
    b. they are used as is and become part of a growing protein
    c. there is a surplus of energy-yielding nutrients
    d. a and c
    e. b and c

23. Which of the following has the highest protein RDA?

    a. a 6 month old infant
    b. a healthy 25 year old female
    c. a 35 year old male
    d. a 30 year old female who exercises frequently

24. What advice would you give to a friend who wants to build bigger muscles?

    a. consume extra protein in the form of foods
    b. engage in rigorous physical training
    c. take an amino acid supplement
    d. a and b
    e. b and c

25. Approximately 7 grams of protein are provided by each of the following foods: **1/2 cup legumes; 1 cup broccoli; 1 ounce cheese; 2 tablespoons peanut butter.** Which of these would be the most nutrient-dense food choice?

    a. 1 cup broccoli
    b. 2 tablespoons peanut butter
    c. 1 ounce cheese
    d. 1/2 cup legumes

ANSWERS

SUMMING UP

(1) nitrogen; (2) amino acids; (3) twenty; (4) shape; (5) essential; (6) peptide; (7) acid; (8) shapes; (9) enzymes; (10) acids; (11) stomach acid; (12) acid; (13) protein; (14) mucus; (15) small intestine; (16) growth; (17) acid-base; (18) carbohydrate; (19) energy; (20) amine; (21) urea; (22) animal; (23) essential; (24) PDCAAS; (25) PER; (26) digested; (27) egg white; (28) tuna fish; (29) body size; (30) children; (31) 0.8; (32) milk; (33) grain; (34) minerals; (35) iron

CHAPTER GLOSSARY

Matching Exercise 1: (1) e; (2) l; (3) c; (4) j; (5) r; (6) h; (7) q; (8) a; (9) n; (10) f; (11) p; (12) i; (13) b; (14) m; (15) k; (16) g; (17) o; (18) d
Matching Exercise 2: (1) p; (2) g; (3) d; (4) k; (5) b; (6) o; (7) l; (8) f; (9) i; (10) m; (11) e; (12) h; (13) a; (14) j; (15) n; (16) c

EXERCISES

Chapter Study Questions:

1. Many poisons are salts of heavy metals which denature proteins whenever they touch them. Milk is given so that the poison will act on the protein of the milk rather than on the protein tissues of the mouth, esophagus, and stomach.

2. Whenever there is not enough energy from carbohydrate or fat; when the diet's protein is low-quality, with too few essential amino acids; when there is too much protein so that not all is needed; when there is too much of any amino acid, such as from a supplement.

3. PDCAAS is geared toward protein to support the maintenance of body tissue of adults, while PER is more suitable to identify the best protein sources to support the rapid growth of infants and children.

4. Legumes are plants of the pea, bean and lentil family which have roots with nodules that contain special bacteria. These bacteria can trap nitrogen from the air in the soil and make it into compounds that become part of the seed. The seeds are rich in high-quality protein compared with those of most other plants.

5. Cooking an egg denatures the protein and makes it more appetizing; in addition, cooking denatures two raw-egg proteins that bind the B vitamin biotin and the mineral iron and slows protein digestion; therefore, cooking eggs liberates biotin and iron and aids digestion.

Short Answer Questions:

1. (a) oxygen; (b) hydrogen; (c) carbon; (d) nitrogen

2. (a) valine; (b) leucine; (c) isoleucine; (d) threonine; (e) lysine; (f) methionine; (g) phenylalanine; (h) tryptophan; (i) histidine

3. (a) used to build proteins; (b) converted to other small nitrogen-containing compounds such as niacin; (c) converted to some other amino acids; (d) converted to glucose; (e) burned as fuel; (f) stored as fat

4. (a) heat; (b) alcohol; (c) acids; (d) bases; (e) salts of heavy metals

5. (a) meat; (b) fish; (c) poultry; (d) cheese; (e) eggs; (f) milk; (g) many soybean products

6. (a) protein efficiency ratio; (b) protein digestibility-corrected amino acid score

7. (a) find body weight in pounds; (b) convert pounds to kilograms; (c) multiply by 0.8 g/kg to find total grams of protein per day

8. (a) meat; (b) milk; (c) vegetable; (d) grain

9. vitamin C; folate

10. vitamin B_{12}; iron

Problem-Solving:

1. 40 grams protein

2.

Menu Item	Grams of Protein
Breakfast	
1 cup skim milk	8
1 boiled egg	7
1 slice whole wheat toast	3
Lunch	
3 oz. hamburger patty	21
1 whole wheat bun	6
tomato and lettuce (1 vegetable serving)	2
2 tsp. mayonnaise	
Dinner	
3 oz. chicken breast	21
1/2 cup green beans	2
1 roll	3
1 cup skim milk	8
	Total: 81

Controversy Questions:

1. Some people do not believe in killing animals for their meat and believe that livestock is treated inhumanely. Others fear contracting diseases, such as mad cow disease, or practice vegetarianism for health reasons.

2. Obesity, diabetes, high blood pressure, heart disease, digestive disorders, and some forms of cancer

3. Vegetarians typically use no tobacco, use alcohol in moderation and may be more physically active.

4. People with colon cancer eat more meat, less fiber, and more saturated fat

5. Calcium, iron, zinc, vitamin D and vitamin B_{12} all require special attention for strict vegetarians.

STUDY AIDS

1. (a) rice; (b) peanut butter; (c) vegetables

2. 2 soybean protein
    3 wheat protein
    1 egg white

SAMPLE TEST ITEMS

1. d (P. 178)
2. a (p. 178)
3. b (p. 179)
4. a (p. 188)
5. a (p. 188)
6. e (p. 189)
7. a (p. 196)
8. d (p. 194)

9. b (p. 192)
10. d (p. 196)
11. b (p. 197-198)
12. a (p. 194)
13. e (p. 195)
14. c (p. 198-199)
15. a (p. 196)
16. d (p. 201)

17. c (p. 201)
18. b (p. 201)
19. e (p. 200)
20. e (p. 181)
21. c (p. 200)
22. d (p. 188)
23. a (p. 194-196)
24. b (p. 183)
25. a (p. 200-201)

CHAPTER 7

The Vitamins

CHAPTER OBJECTIVES

After completing this chapter, you should be able to:

1. Define the term vitamin and explain how vitamins are classified.

2. Describe the characteristics of fat-soluble vitamins and water-soluble vitamins and explain how they differ.

3. List the chief functions and food sources of each vitamin and describe any major deficiency and toxicity symptoms associated with each.

4. Identify groups of people who may benefit from a multinutrient supplement and discuss guidelines for choosing an appropriate supplement.

5. Describe the best method of planning a diet that is rich in vitamins.

6. Discuss the evidence suggesting that antioxidant nutrients and phytochemicals protect against cancer, heart disease, and age-related blindness. (Controversy 7)

KEY CONCEPTS

✓ Vitamins are essential, noncaloric nutrients, needed in tiny amounts in the diet, that help to drive cell processes. The fat-soluble vitamins are vitamins A, D, E, and K; the water-soluble vitamins are the B vitamins and vitamin C.

✓ Vitamin A is essential to vision, integrity of epithelial tissue, bone growth, reproduction, and more. Vitamin A deficiency causes blindness, sickness, and death and is a major problem worldwide. Overdoses are possible and cause many serious symptoms. Foods are preferable to supplements for supplying vitamin A.

✓ The vitamin A precursor in plants, beta-carotene, is an effective antioxidant in the body. Brightly colored plant foods are richest in beta-carotene, and diets containing these foods are associated with eye health.

✓ Vitamin D raises mineral levels in the blood, notably calcium and phosphorus, permitting bone formation and maintenance. A deficiency can cause rickets in childhood or osteomalacia in later life. Vitamin D is the most toxic of all the vitamins, and excesses are dangerous or deadly. People exposed to the sun make vitamin D from a cholesterol-like compound in their skin; fortified milk is an important food source.

✓ Vitamin E acts as an antioxidant in cell membranes and is especially important for the integrity of cells that are constantly exposed to high oxygen concentrations, namely, the lungs and blood cells, both red and white. Vitamin E deficiency is rare in human beings, but it does occur in newborn premature infants. The vitamin is widely distributed in plant foods; it is destroyed by high heat; toxicity is rare.

✓ Vitamin K is necessary for blood to clot; deficiency causes uncontrolled bleeding. The bacterial inhabitants of the digestive tract produce vitamin K, but the extent to which the body uses this intestinal vitamin K has not been determined.

✓ As part of coenzymes, the B vitamins help enzymes do their jobs.

✓ The B vitamins facilitate the work of every cell. Some help generate energy; others help make protein and new cells. B vitamins work everywhere in the body tissue to metabolize carbohydrate, fat, and protein.

✓ Every cell is affected by a B vitamin deficiency. Deficiencies of single B vitamins are rare; a person deficient in one is likely to be deficient in others.

✓ Historically, famous B vitamin-deficiency diseases are beriberi (thiamin), pellagra (niacin), and pernicious anemia (vitamin B_{12}). Pellagra can be prevented by adequate protein because the amino acid tryptophan can be converted to niacin in the body. A high intake of folate can mask the blood symptom of vitamin B_{12}, deficiency but will not prevent the associated nerve damage. Vitamin B_6 is important in amino acid metabolism and can be toxic in excess. Biotin and pantothenic acid are important to the body and are abundant in food.

✓ Choline is needed in the diet, but it is not a vitamin and deficiencies are unheard of outside of the laboratory. Many other substances that people claim are B vitamins are not. Among these substances are carnitine, inositol, and lipoic acid.

✓ Vitamin C, an antioxidant, helps to maintain the connective tissue protein collagen, protects against infection, and helps in iron absorption. The theory that vitamin C prevents or cures colds or cancer is not well supported by research. Taking high vitamin C doses may be unwise. Ample vitamin C can be obtained from foods.

✓ People who routinely fail to obtain the recommended amounts of vitamins and minerals from the diet and people with special needs, such as those who are pregnant or elderly, may be at risk for deficiencies and may benefit from a multivitamin-mineral supplement.

✓ Before you decide to take supplements, make sure to recognize the potential for toxicity.

✓ Ingredients of dietary supplements are not tested or approved by the FDA before marketing, but their labels must meet certain criteria.

✓ If you decide to take a supplement, examine the ingredients on supplement labels and choose one that satisfies your needs.

SUMMING UP

A vitamin is defined as an essential, noncaloric, organic nutrient needed in (1) _____

amounts in the diet. The role of many vitamins is to help make possible the processes by which

other nutrients are digested, (2) _____, and metabolized, or built into body

(3) _____. Some of the vitamins occur in foods in a form known as

(4) _____, or provitamins. The vitamins fall naturally into two classes including

the (5) _____ soluble vitamins and the (6) _____ soluble vitamins.

Vitamin A plays parts in such diverse functions as (7) _____,

maintenance of skin and body linings, bone growth and reproduction. One of the active forms of

vitamin A is (8) _____, which is stored in the liver. In plants, vitamin A exists

only in its precursor forms; the most abundant of these is (9) _____. Rich food

sources of beta carotene include carrots, sweet potatoes, pumpkins, mango, (10) _____,

and apricots, as well as dark green vegetables.

Vitamin D is one member of a team of nutrients and hormones that maintains blood

calcium and phosphorus levels and thereby (11) _____ integrity. The vitamin D

deficiency disease in (12) _____ is called rickets, while the comparable disease

in adults is referred to as (13)_____. Vitamin D is the most potentially

The Vitamins

(14) _____ of all vitamins and as little as 5 times the recommended amount have

been associated with signs of Vitamin D toxicity.   People can make vitamin D from a

(15) _____ compound whenever the sun shines on their skin. The recommended

intake for vitamin D is (16) _____ micrograms per day for adults 19 to 50 years.

Vitamin E is like a bodyguard for other substances and it serves as an

(17) _____. In the body, it exerts an especially important antioxidant effect in

the (18) _____. Conditions that cause malabsorption of (19) _____

can cause vitamin E deficiencies, although vitamin E deficiency is rare in most situations. The

DRI intake recommendation for vitamin E is (20) _____ milligrams a day for

adults. About 20% of the vitamin E people consume comes from (21) _____

oils and products made from them.

Vitamin K is the fat-soluble vitamin necessary for the synthesis of proteins involved in

(22) _____. It can be obtained from the nonfood source of (23) _____

bacteria. However, vitamin K deficiencies may occur in newborn infants and people who have

taken (24) _____ that have killed their intestinal bacteria.

The B vitamins and vitamin C are known together as the (25) _____

vitamins. The B vitamins act as part of (26) _____. Niacin, thiamin and

riboflavin participate in the energy   (27) _____ of every body cell. For

(28) _____, which is tied closely to amino acid metabolism, the amount needed

is proportional to (29) _____ intake. The thiamin deficiency disease is called

(30) _____, while the (31) _____ deficiency disease is known

as pellagra. In the body, the amino acid (32) _____ is converted to niacin. Strict

vegetarians are most apt to be deficient in (33) _____. The vitamin C deficiency

disease is scurvy, which can be prevented by an intake of (34) _____ milligrams of

vitamin C per day. However, the adult DRI intake recommendation for vitamin C is

(35) _____ milligrams for men and 75 milligrams for women.

CHAPTER GLOSSARY

Matching Exercise 1:

_____ 1. biotin

_____ 2. vitamin B_6

_____ 3. rickets

_____ 4. erythrocyte hemolysis

_____ 5. choline

_____ 6. pellagra

_____ 7. scurvy

_____ 8. night blindness

_____ 9. prooxidant

_____ 10. niacin

_____ 11. riboflavin

_____ 12. vitamin B_{12}

_____ 13. inositol

_____ 14. ascorbic acid

_____ 15. beriberi

_____ 16. pernicious anemia

_____ 17. folate

_____ 18. thiamin

_____ 19. carotenoid

_____ 20. osteomalacia

a. the vitamin C-deficiency disease

b. a nonessential nutrient found in cell membranes

c. a B vitamin needed in protein metabolism; its three active forms are pyridoxine, pyridoxal, and pyridoxamine

d. a B vitamin needed in energy metabolism; it can be eaten preformed or can be made in the body from tryptophan

e. a B vitamin that acts as part of a coenzyme important in the manufacture of new cells

f. rupture of the red blood cells, caused by vitamin E deficiency

g. the thiamin-deficiency disease

h. a B vitamin; a coenzyme necessary for fat synthesis and other metabolic reactions

i. one of the active forms of vitamin C

j. the niacin-deficiency disease

k. a B vitamin active in the body's energy-release mechanisms

l. the vitamin D-deficiency disease in children

m. slow recovery of vision after exposure to flashes of bright light at night; an early symptom of vitamin A deficiency

n. a B vitamin that helps convert folate to its active form and also helps maintain the sheaths around nerve cells

o. a compound that triggers reactions involving oxygen

p. a nonessential nutrient used to make the phospholipid lecithin and other molecules

q. a vitamin B_{12}-deficiency disease, caused by lack of intrinsic factor and characterized by large, immature red blood cells and damage to the nervous system

r. a B vitamin involved in the body's use of fuels

s. the vitamin D deficiency disease in adults

t. any of a type of pigments in foods ranging from light yellow to reddish orange

The Vitamins

Matching Exercise 2:

_____ 1. collagen

_____ 2. IU

_____ 3. xerosis

_____ 4. rhodopsin

_____ 5. tocopherol

_____ 6. cornea

_____ 7. xerophthalmia

_____ 8. RAE

_____ 9. macular degeneration

_____ 10. coenzyme

_____ 11. beta-carotene

_____ 12. precursors

_____ 13. intrinsic factor

_____ 14. retinol

_____ 15. keratin

_____ 16. retina

_____ 17. vitamins

_____ 18. epithelial tissue

_____ 19. homocysteine

a. the layer of light-sensitive nerve cells lining the back of the inside of the eye

b. a kind of alcohol

c. a small molecule that works with an enzyme to promote the enzyme's activity

d. the chief protein of most connective tissues, including scars, ligaments, and tendons, and the underlying matrix on which bones and teeth are built

e. a factor found inside a system

f. a new measure of vitamin A activity of beta-carotene and other vitamin A precursors

g. organic compounds that are vital to life and indispensable to body functions, but are needed only in minute amounts

h. a measure of fat-soluble vitamin activity sometimes used on supplement labels

i. a common, progressive loss of function of the part of the retina that is most crucial to focused vision; often leads to blindness

j. compounds that can be converted into active vitamins

k. the light-sensitive pigment of the cells in the retina

l. the normal protein of hair and nails

m. hardening of the cornea of the eye in advanced vitamin A deficiency that can lead to blindness

n. an orange pigment with antioxidant activity; a vitamin A precursor made by plants and stored in human fat tissue

o. the hard, transparent membrane covering the outside of the eye

p. one of the active forms of vitamin A made from beta-carotene in animal and human bodies

q. drying of the cornea; a symptom of vitamin A deficiency

r. the layers of the body that serve as selective barriers to environmental factors

s. an amino acid produced as an intermediate compound during amino acid metabolism

EXERCISES

Answer these chapter study questions:

1. List the general characteristics of fat-soluble vitamins.

2. Do individuals have to eat vitamin D to have enough in their bodies? Why or why not?

3. Name three reasons why it is almost impossible to create vitamin E deficiencies in humans.

4. Why would someone who had part of the stomach removed develop deficiency symptoms for vitamin B_{12}?

5. Is it possible for a person consuming adequate protein and adequate calories to be deficient in niacin? Why or why not?

Complete these short answer questions:

1. The fat-soluble vitamins include:

    a.
    b.
    c.
    d.

2. Vitamin A has parts to play in such diverse functions as:

    a.
    b.
    c.
    d.
    e.
    f.

3. The richest food sources of beta carotene include:

    a.
    b.
    c.
    d.
    e.
    f.
    g.
    h.

4. The earliest symptoms of vitamin A overdoses are:

    a.
    b.
    c.
    d.
    e.
    f.

5. To raise the level of blood calcium, the body can draw from these places:

    a.
    b.
    c.

6. Vitamin K's richest plant sources are:

    a.
    b.

7. Significant food sources of vitamin D include:

    a.
    b.
    c.

8. In adults, vitamin E deficiency is usually associated with diseases of these organs:

    a.
    b.
    c.

9. The best sources of folate are _____ vegetables and fruits.

10. In the U.S. today, scurvy may be seen in these groups:

    a.
    b.
    c.

Solve these problems:

1. Your friend is taking supplements of the antioxidant nutrients in an effort to reduce her risk of cancer. Based on the latest research in this area, what advice would you offer your friend?

2. If a person consumed a diet composed of 1200 micrograms of beta-carotene from food, how many micrograms of retinol would this supply in the body?

Solve these controversy questions:

1. What are free radicals? Are they all bad?

2. What are the body's two main systems of defense against damage from free radicals?

3. What is the primary characteristic of the diet of populations with high cancer rates?

4. Why did the FDA reject a request by the supplement industry to allow health claims on the labels of antioxidant supplements?

5. What is the relationship between carotenoids and macular degeneration?

STUDY AIDS

1. Complete the following chart which identifies names, chief functions, deficiency disease names, and major food sources of some of the fat-soluble and water-soluble vitamins.

Name	Chief Functions	Deficiency Disease Name(s)	Food Sources
A	_____ bone_____ reproduction _____cells	hypovitaminosis A	For retinol: fortified_____ or _____ cheese _____ or cream eggs _____ For beta-carotene: dark leafy greens deep orange fruits and _____
D	mineralization of_____	rickets _____	_____milk eggs liver _____
E	_____ protects PUFA and vitamin_____	no name	polyunsaturated plant_____ _____germ vegetables
K	synthesis of blood_____ proteins	no name	liver _____type vegetables green_____ vegetables milk
Thiamin	part of a _____ used in energy metabolism	_____	occurs in all nutritious foods

Riboflavin	part of a coenzyme used in_____ metabolism	_____	milk, yogurt and cottage cheese
			_____ leafy green vegetables whole grain or _____ breads and _____
Niacin	part of a _____ used in energy metabolism	_____	milk _____ meat _____ fish enriched _____ and cereals all _____- containing foods
Vitamin C	_____synthesis _____ thyroxine synthesis _____acid metabolism	_____	_____fruits _____-type vegetables dark green _____ canteloupe _____ peppers lettuce _____ potatoes _____ or _____

2.   Use the following table in your textbook as a study aid: Table 7-2 on page 240.

SAMPLE TEST ITEMS

Comprehension Level Items:

1.   The vitamins fall naturally into _____ classes.

     a.   two
     b.   three
     c.   four
     d.   five

2.   All of the following are characteristics of fat-soluble vitamins *except*:

     a.   they require bile for absorption
     b.   they can reach toxic levels
     c.   they are easily excreted
     d.   they are stored in fatty tissues

3. The first fat-soluble vitamin to be recognized was vitamin:

   a. D
   b. K
   c. E
   d. A

4. A vitamin A precursor found in plants is:

   a. called beta carotene
   b. a bright orange color
   c. yellow in color
   d. a and b
   e. a and c

5. All of the following are good sources of beta carotene *except*:

   a. carrots
   b. pumpkins
   c. sweet corn
   d. apricots

6. The vitamin D deficiency disease in children is known as:

   a. osteodystrophy
   b. rickets
   c. pellagra
   d. osteomalacia

7. People who are exposed to the sun make vitamin D from:

   a. cholesterol
   b. carotene
   c. polyunsaturated fats
   d. saturated fats

8. Vitamin E exerts an especially important antioxidant effect in the:

   a. kidneys
   b. heart
   c. lungs
   d. stomach

9. The DRI for vitamin E is _____ milligrams a day for adults.

   a. 5
   b. 8
   c. 10
   d. 15

10. Vitamin K deficiencies may occur in:

    a.   newborn infants
    b.   people who have undergone surgery
    c.   people who have taken antibiotics
    d.   a and c
    e.   b and c

11. The niacin deficiency disease is known as:

    a.   osteomalacia
    b.   scurvy
    c.   pellagra
    d.   beriberi

12. A high intake of _____ can mask the anemia caused by vitamin B_{12} deficiency.

    a.   thiamin
    b.   folate
    c.   riboflavin
    d.   niacin

13. What is the amount of vitamin C required to prevent the symptoms of scurvy from appearing?

    a.   10 milligrams
    b.   20 milligrams
    c.   30 milligrams
    d.   40 milligrams

14. The amount needed of this vitamin is proportional to protein intake:

    a.   thiamin
    b.   riboflavin
    c.   niacin
    d.   vitamin B_6

15. People addicted to alcohol may develop a deficiency of:

    a.   niacin
    b.   thiamin
    c.   vitamin B_6
    d.   vitamin B_{12}

16. Vitamin B_{12} is present only in:

    a.   grains
    b.   plants
    c.   animals
    d.   vegetables

17. In the U.S. today, scurvy has been found in all of the following *except*:

    a. breast-fed infants
    b. infants fed only cow's milk
    c. elderly
    d. people addicted to drugs

18. Which of the following supplements would be the most appropriate to choose?

    a. one that comes in a chewable form
    b. one that provides all the vitamins and minerals in amounts smaller than or close to the intake recommendations
    c. one that provides more than the DRI recommended intake for vitamin A, vitamin D and minerals
    d. one that provides more than the Tolerable Upper Intake Level for any nutrient

19. Vitamin C supplements in any dosage may be dangerous for people with an overload of _____ in the blood.

    a. zinc
    b. calcium
    c. magnesium
    d. iron

Application Level Items:

20. A friend of yours complains that she is unable to see for a short period of time after she encounters a flash of bright light at night. Which of the following statements would you make to your friend?

    a. your eyes are probably well nourished and normal
    b. you are suffering from vitamin A deficiency
    c. you have night blindness
    d. you may need to check your diet for vitamin A deficiency

21. A couple you know gives their infant a jar of baby carrots to eat every day. This child runs the risk of:

    a. developing an allergic reaction to carrots
    b. developing a vitamin A toxicity
    c. having his skin turn bright yellow
    d. a and b
    e. b and c

22. Which of the following would have the lowest need for vitamin A?

    a. a man
    b. a child
    c. a woman
    d. a lactating woman

23. You have a friend who has been experiencing appetite loss, nausea, vomiting, and increased urination and thirst. A medical examination reveals that calcium has been deposited in the heart and kidneys. Based on these symptoms you suspect that your friend has been taking supplements of:

    a. vitamin A
    b. vitamin K
    c. vitamin D
    d. vitamin E

24. Which of the following would ***not*** be at risk for developing a vitamin D deficiency?

    a. a woman who is institutionalized
    b. a man who works the night shift for several years
    c. a dark-skinned child who lives in a northern city
    d. an adult who eats cereal with milk for breakfast every day

25. An athlete who consumes a high protein diet would have an increased need for:

    a. vitamin B_6
    b. vitamin C
    c. vitamin B_{12}
    d. thiamin

ANSWERS

SUMMING UP

(1) tiny; (2) absorbed; (3) structures; (4) precursors; (5) fat; (6) water; (7) vision; (8) retinol; (9) beta carotene; (10) cantaloupe: (11) bone; (12) children; (13) osteomalacia; (14) toxic; (15) cholesterol; (16) 5; (17) antioxidant; (18) lungs; (19) fat; (20) 15; (21) vegetable; (22) blood clotting; (23) intestinal; (24) antibiotics; (25) water-soluble; (26) coenzymes; (27) metabolism; (28) vitamin B_6; (29) protein; (30) beriberi; (31) niacin; (32) tryptophan; (33) vitamin B_{12}; (34) 10; (35) 90

CHAPTER GLOSSARY

Matching Exercise 1: (1) h; (2) c; (3) l; (4) f; (5) p; (6) j; (7) a; (8) m; (9) o; (10) d; (11) k; (12) n; (13) b; (14) i; (15) g; (16) q; (17) e; (18) r; (19) t; (20) s.
Matching Exercise 2: (1) d; (2) h; (3) q; (4) k; (5) b; (6) o; (7) m; (8) f; (9) i; (10) c; (11) n; (12) j; (13) e; (14) p; (15) l; (16) a; (17) g; (18) r; (19) s.

EXERCISES

Chapter Study Questions:

1. They require bile for absorption. They generally occur together in the fats and oils of foods; once they have been absorbed from the intestinal tract, they are stored in the liver and fatty tissues until the body needs them; excesses can reach toxic levels; they can be lost from the digestive tract with undigested fat.

2. Humans do not have to eat vitamin D because they can make it from a cholesterol compound whenever ultraviolet light from the sun shines on their skin. The compound is transformed into a vitamin D precursor and is absorbed directly into the blood.

3. Because vitamin E is so widespread in food it is almost impossible to create a vitamin E deficient diet. In addition, the body stores so much vitamin E in its fatty tissues that a person could not keep on eating a vitamin E free diet for long enough to deplete those stores and produce a deficiency. Finally, the cells may recycle their working supply of vitamin E, using the same molecules over and over.

4. The absorption of vitamin B_{12} requires an intrinsic factor, which is synthesized in the stomach. When part of the stomach has been removed, it cannot produce enough of the intrinsic factor. Without enough of the intrinsic factor, the person cannot absorb the vitamin even though he may be getting enough in the diet.

5. A person eating adequate protein will not be deficient in niacin because the amino acid tryptophan is converted to niacin in the body.

Short Answer Questions:

1. (a) A; (b) D; (c) E; (d) K

2. (a) vision; (b) maintenance of body linings and skin; (c) bone and body growth; (d) reproduction; (e) normal cell development; (f) immune defenses

3. (a) carrots; (b) sweet potatoes; (c) pumpkins; (d) cantaloupe; (e) apricots; (f) spinach; (g) broccoli; (h) mango

4. (a) blurred vision; (b) growth failure in children; (c) loss of appetite; (d) headache; (e) itching of skin; (f) irritability

5. (a) bones; (b) food in the digestive tract; (c) kidneys, which recycle calcium

6. (a) dark-green leafy vegetables; (b) members of the cabbage family

7. (a) butter; (b) cream; (c) fortified margarine

8. (a) liver; (b) gallbladder; (c) pancreas

9. uncooked

10. (a) infants fed only cow's milk; (b) elderly; (c) people addicted to alcohol or other drugs

Problem-Solving:

1. Research findings thus far do not support taking antioxidant supplements to prevent cancer. More research is needed to quantify them and to clarify the risks and benefits. However, there is strong support for recommendations to increase consumption of fruits and vegetables to provide these nutrients.

2. 100 micrograms of retinol

Controversy Questions:

1. Free radicals are atoms or molecules with one or more unpaired electrons that make the atom or molecule unstable and highly reactive; they are not all bad because their destructive properties are put to good use by some cells of the immune system.

2. Its reserves of antioxidants and its enzyme systems that oppose oxidation.

3. They consume few vegetables and fruits, especially those containing beta-carotene and other carotenoids.

4. Because, after reviewing the evidence, the agency concluded that diets high in fruits and vegetables, which are particularly good sources of beta-carotene and vitamin C, are strongly associated with reduced risk of several types of cancer; reductions in risk could not be attributed solely to the named vitamins.

5. Carotenoids are believed to filter out damaging light rays before they can harm the macula and they may improve visual abilities.

STUDY AIDS

Name	Chief Functions	Deficiency Disease Name(s)	Food Sources
A	**vision** bone **growth** reproduction **epithelial** cells	hypovitaminosis A	*For retinol:* fortified **milk** or **margarine** cheese **butter** or cream eggs **liver** *For beta-carotene:* dark leafy greens deep orange fruits and **vegetables**
D	mineralization of **bones**	rickets **osteomalacia**	**fortified** milk eggs liver **sardines**

E	**antioxidant** protects PUFA and vitamin **A**	no name	polyunsaturated plant **oils** **wheat** germ vegetables
K	synthesis of blood **clotting** proteins	no name	liver **cabbage**-type vegetables green **leafy** vegetables milk
Thiamin	part of a **coenzyme** used in energy metabolism	**beriberi**	occurs in all nutritious foods
Riboflavin	part of a coenzyme used in **energy** metabolism	**ariboflavinosis**	milk, yogurt and cottage cheese **meat** leafy green vegetables whole grain or **enriched** breads and **cereals**
Niacin	part of a **coenzyme** used in energy metabolism	**pellagra**	milk **eggs** meat **poultry** fish enriched **breads** and cereals all **protein**-containing foods
Vitamin C	**collagen** synthesis **antioxidant** thyroxine synthesis **amino** acid metabolism	**scurvy**	**citrus** fruits **cabbage**-type vegetables dark green **vegetables** canteloupe **strawberries** peppers lettuce **tomatoes** potatoes **papayas** or **mangos**

SAMPLE TEST ITEMS

1. a (p. 212)
2. c (p. 213)
3. d (p. 213)
4. d (p. 213)
5. c (p. 217)
6. b (p. 218)
7. a (p. 219)
8. c (p. 221)

9. d (p. 222)
10. d (p. 223)
11. c (p. 228)
12. b (p. 230-233)
13. a (p. 237)
14. d (p. 234)
15. b (p. 227-228)
16. c (p. 232)

17. a (p. 237)
18. b (p. 243-244)
19. d (p. 237)
20. a (p. 213-214)
21. c (p. 217)
22. b (p. 216)
23. c (p. 219)
24. d (p. 220)
25. a (p. 234)

CHAPTER 8

Water and Minerals

CHAPTER OBJECTIVES

After completing this chapter, you should be able to:

1. Discuss the major roles of water in the body and the amount of water needed by adults.

2. Describe how the body regulates water intake and excretion to maintain water balance.

3. Compare the arguments for and against drinking bottled water.

4. Explain the role of minerals in maintaining the body's fluid and electrolyte balance and acid-base balance.

5. List the major roles and important deficiency and toxicity symptoms for each major and trace mineral.

6. List good food sources for the major and trace elements.

7. Discuss the lifestyle choices that reduce the risk of osteoporosis. (Controversy 8)

KEY CONCEPTS

✓ Water acts as a solvent, provides the medium for transportation, participates in chemical reactions, provides lubrication and shock protection, and aids in temperature regulation in the human body.

✓ Water makes up about 60 percent of the body's weight A change in the body's water content can bring a change in body weight.

✓ Water losses from the body necessitate intake equal to output to maintain balance. The brain regulates water intake; the brain and kidneys regulate water excretion. Dehydration can have serious consequences.

✓ Many factors influence a person's need for water. The water of beverages and foods helps meet water needs, as does the water formed during cellular breakdown of energy nutrients.

✓ Hard water is high in calcium and magnesium. Soft water is high in sodium, and it dissolves cadmium and lead from pipes.

✓ Electrolytes help keep fluids in their proper compartments and buffer these fluids, permitting all life processes to take place.

✓ Calcium makes up bone and tooth structure and plays roles in nerve transmission, muscle contraction, and blood clotting. Calcium absorption rises when there is a dietary deficiency or an increased need such as during growth.

✓ Most of the phosphorus in the body is in the bones and teeth. Phosphorus helps maintain acid-base balance, is part of the genetic material in cells, assists in energy metabolism, and forms part of cell membranes. Under normal circumstances, deficiencies of phosphorus are unknown.

✓ Most of the body's magnesium is in the bones and can be drawn out for all the cells to use in building protein and using energy. Most people in the United States fail to obtain enough magnesium from their food.

✓ Sodium is the main positively charged ion outside the body's cells. Sodium attracts water. Thus, too much sodium (or salt) may aggravate hypertension. Diets rarely lack sodium.

✓ Potassium, the major positive ion inside cells, is important in many metabolic functions. Fresh foods are the best sources of potassium. Diuretics can deplete the body's potassium and so can be dangerous; potassium excess can also be dangerous.

✓ Chloride is the body's major negative ion; it is responsible for stomach acidity and assists in maintaining proper body chemistry.

✓ Sulfur plays important roles in body proteins.

✓ Iodine is part of the hormone thyroxine, which influences energy metabolism. The deficiency diseases are goiter and cretinism. Iodine occurs naturally in seafood and in foods grown on land that was once covered by oceans; it is an additive in milk and bakery products. Large amounts are poisonous.

✓ Most iron in the body is contained in hemoglobin and myoglobin or occurs as part of enzymes in the energy-yielding pathways. Iron-deficiency anemia is a problem worldwide; too much iron is toxic. Iron is lost through menstruation and other bleeding; reduced absorption and the shedding of intestinal cells protect against overload. For maximum iron absorption, use meat, other iron sources, and vitamin C together.

✓ Zinc assists enzymes in all cells. Deficiencies in children cause growth retardation with sexual immaturity. Zinc supplements can reach toxic doses, but zinc in foods is non-toxic. Animal foods are the best sources.

✓ Selenium works with an enzyme system to protect body compounds from oxidation. A deficiency induces a disease of the heart. Deficiencies are rare in developed countries, but toxicities occur from overuse of supplements.

✓ Fluoride stabilizes bones and makes teeth resistant to decay. Excess fluoride discolors teeth; large doses are toxic.

✓ Chromium works with the hormone insulin to control blood glucose concentrations. Chromium is present in a variety of unrefined foods.

✓ Copper is needed to form hemoglobin and collagen and assists in many other body processes. Copper deficiency is rare.

✓ Many different trace elements play important roles in the body. All of the trace minerals are toxic in excess.

SUMMING UP

Water makes up about (1) _____ percent of all the body's weight and is the most

indispensable nutrient of all. Thirst and (2) _____ govern water intake, although

(3) _____ lags behind a lack of water. Water excretion is governed by the brain

and the (4) _____. A change in the body's water content can bring a change in

body (5) _____. Water losses from the body necessitate intake of an equal

amount of (6) _____ to maintain (7) _____. In the body, water

provides the medium for (8) _____, chemical reactions, shock protection,

lubrication, and (9) _____ regulation.

Under normal dietary and environmental conditions adults should consume between 1

and 1 1/2 milliliters of water for each (10) _____ spent in the day. For the person

who expends about 2,000 calories a day, this works out to be about (11) _____ liters. Hard water is high in calcium and (12) _____, while soft water is high in (13) _____.

Most of the body's water weight is contained inside the (14) _____, and some water also bathes the (15) _____ of the cells. Body cells can pump (16) _____ across their membranes, but not water, and these minerals attract the water to come along with them. The cells use minerals for this purpose in a special form, known as ions or (17) _____. The result of the system's working properly is (18) _____ and electrolyte balance. The minerals also help manage another balancing act, the (19) _____ balance. Among the major minerals, some, when dissolved in water, give rise to acids, and some to (20) _____.

Calcium is by far the most (21) _____ mineral in the body. Calcium makes up bone and (22) _____ structure and plays roles in (23) _____ transmission, muscle contraction and blood clotting. Adult bone loss is called (24) _____. The DRI recommended intake for calcium has been set at (25) _____ milligrams for adolescents.

Sodium is the chief ion used to maintain the volume of fluid (26) _____ cells and it contributes (27) _____ percent of the weight of the compound sodium chloride. Sodium helps maintain (28) _____ balance and is essential to nerve transmission and muscle contraction. It is widespread in foods and should be consumed in (29) _____ .

Both potassium deficiency and excess can be dangerous and (30) _____ can deplete body potassium. Other major minerals include (31) _____, which helps strands of protein to assume and hold a functional shape, magnesium, phosphorus and (32) _____, which is part of the stomach's hydrochloric acid.

One of the trace minerals is iodine, which is part of the hormone (33) _____, which regulates the basal metabolic rate. Every living cell contains (34) _____, which is contained in hemoglobin and (35) _____.

Zinc works with proteins in every organ as a helper for more than 50 (36) _____

and is found primarily in animal foods. Fluoride stabilizes bone and makes (37) _____

resistant to decay.

CHAPTER GLOSSARY

Matching Exercise 1:

_____ 1. hemoglobin

_____ 2. osteoporosis

_____ 3. fluid and electrolyte balance

_____ 4. goiter

_____ 5. phytates

_____ 6. peak bone mass

_____ 7. iron overload

_____ 8. buffers

_____ 9. tannins

_____ 10. heme

_____ 11. dehydration

_____ 12. iron deficiency

_____ 13. hydroxyapatite

_____ 14. cretinism

_____ 15. MFP factor

_____ 16. acid-base balance

_____ 17. myoglobin

_____ 18. pica

a. compounds in tea (especially black tea), and coffee that bind iron

b. enlargement of the thyroid gland due to iodine deficiency

c. the oxygen-holding protein of the muscles

d. the highest attainable bone density for an individual

e. the oxygen-carrying protein of the blood

f. severe mental and physical retardation of an infant caused by the mother's iodine deficiency during her pregnancy

g. maintenance of the proper amounts and kinds of fluids and minerals in each compartment of the body

h. the condition of having depleted iron stores, which, at the extreme, causes iron-deficiency anemia

i. maintenance of the proper degree of acidity in each of the body's fluids

j. a reduction of the bone mass of older persons in which the bones become porous and fragile

k. molecules that can help to keep the pH of a solution from changing by gathering or releasing H ions

l. the chief crystal of bone, formed from calcium and phosphorus

m. loss of water

n. a craving for nonfood substances

o. the state of having more iron in the body than it needs or can handle; too much iron is toxic and can damage the liver

p. a factor (identity unknown) present in meat, fish, and poultry that enhances the absorption of nonheme iron present in the same foods or in other foods eaten at the same time

q. the iron-containing portion of the hemoglobin and myoglobin molecules

r. compounds present in plant foods (particularly whole grains) that bind iron and prevent its absorption

---

Matching Exercise 2:

_____ 1. soft water

_____ 2. fluorapatite

_____ 3. acquifers

_____ 4. fluorosis

_____ 5. hard water

_____ 6. minerals

_____ 7. ions

_____ 8. major minerals

_____ 9. trace minerals

_____ 10. salts

_____ 11. surface water

_____ 12. water balance

_____ 13. ground water

_____ 14. diuretics

_____ 15. electrolytes

_____ 16. water intoxication

_____ 17. leavened

_____ 18. hypertension

a. compounds, usually medications, causing increased urinary water excretion
b. water with high calcium and magnesium concentrations
c. compounds composed of charged particles
d. the rare condition in which body water content is too high
e. electrically charged particles, such as sodium (positively charged) or chloride (negatively charged)
f. water with a high sodium concentration
g. water that comes from underground aquifers
h. underground rock formations containing water that can be drawn to the surface for use
i. the balance between water intake and water excretion, which keeps the body's water content constant
j. essential mineral nutrients found in the human body in amounts larger than 5 grams
k. compounds that partly dissociate in water to form ions, such as the potassium ion (K+) and the chloride ion (Cl-)
l. a crystal of bones and teeth, formed when fluoride displaces the hydroxy portion of hydroxyapatite
m. water that comes from lakes, rivers and reservoirs
n. naturally occurring, inorganic, homogenous substances; chemical elements
o. essential mineral nutrients found in the human body in amounts less than 5 grams
p. discoloration of the teeth due to ingestion of too much fluoride during tooth development
q. high blood pressure
r. literally, "*lightened*" by yeast cells, which digest some carbohydrate components of the dough and leave behind bubbles of gas that make the bread rise

EXERCISES

Answer these chapter study questions:

1. Discuss the health implications of drinking hard water versus soft water.

2. Why is setting recommended intakes for calcium difficult?

3. Why are recommended intakes for calcium higher for young people and for those in old age?

4. Why should someone taking diuretics, which cause potassium loss, be advised to eat potassium-rich foods?

5. Define the term *pica*. What type of mineral deficiency is associated with pica?

Complete these short answer questions:

1. The major minerals include:

    a.
    b.
    c.
    d.
    e.
    f.
    g.

2. The distinction between hard water and soft water is based on these three minerals:

    a.
    b.
    c.

3. The major roles of calcium in the body's fluids include:

    a.

    b.

    c.

    d.

    e.

    f.

4. All of the following can deplete the body of needed sodium:

    a.
    b.
    c.
    d.

5. The person who wishes to learn to control salt intake should:

    a.
    b.

6. Deficiency of magnesium may occur as a result of:

    a.
    b.
    c.
    d.
    e.

7. The need for iodine is easily met by consuming:

    a.
    b.

8. Factors that hinder iron absorption include:

    a.
    b.
    c.

Solve these problems:

Modify the following recipe to make it lower in calories, fat, and sodium and to substitute polyunsaturated fat for saturated fat.

Chicken Pot Pie

Pastry
1 cup flour
1/4 tsp. salt
2 tbsp. water
1/3 cup lard

Filling

1/3 cup chopped potatoes
1/3 cup sliced carrots
1/3 cup canned green peas
1/4 cup chopped celery
1 tbsp. chopped onion
1/2 cup boiling water
1/4 cup butter
1/4 cup flour
1/2 tsp. salt
1/8 tsp. pepper
1/8 tsp. poultry seasoning
1 1/3 cup chicken broth
2/3 cup cream
1 1/2 cup diced, cooked chicken

Modifications: _____

_____

_____

Solve these controversy questions:

1. Differentiate between trabecular bone and cortical bone.

2. What are environmental factors currently under study for their roles in lowering bone density?

3. How is genetics thought to influence bone density?

4. What types of physical activity are recommended for building muscle and bone strength to reduce the risk of osteoporosis?

5. Why should calcium supplements be taken in low doses several times a day versus a large dose all at once?

STUDY AIDS

1. Complete the following chart which identifies the names, chief functions, deficiency disease names, and major food sources of some of the major and trace minerals.

Major Minerals

Name	Chief Functions	Deficiency Disease Name	Food Sources
Calcium	makes up bone and _____structure normal muscle contraction nerve functioning blood_____ immune defenses	_____	milk small_____ with bones tofu greens legumes
Magnesium	_____mineralization building of protein normal muscle contraction transmission of nerve_____ maintenance of _____		nuts _____ whole grains dark green_____ seafoods _____ cocoa
Sodium	maintains normal fluid balance maintains normal _____balance		salt _____foods _____sauce

133

Trace Minerals

Name	Chief Functions	Deficiency Disease Name	Food Sources
Iron	part of the protein _____	_____	_____meats
	part of the protein myoglobin necessary for utilization of_____ in the body		poultry shellfish eggs legumes _____fruits
Iodine	component of thyroid hormone _____	_____ _____	_____ _____salt bread
Zinc	part of insulin and many_____ normal _____ development		_____-containing foods

2. Use the following tables in your textbook as study aids: Table 8-4 on page 277; Table 8-5 on page 281; Table 8-8 on page 289.

SAMPLE TEST ITEMS

Comprehension Level Items:

1. The distinction between the major and trace minerals means that:

   a. the major minerals are more important than the trace minerals
   b. the major minerals play more important roles than the trace minerals
   c. the major minerals are present in larger quantities than the trace minerals
   d. a and c
   e. b and c

2. All of the following play a role in water intake *except*:

   a. the mouth
   b. the volume of blood
   c. the hypothalamus
   d. the lungs

3. One of the principal minerals in hard water is:

    a. calcium
    b. fluoride
    c. sodium
    d. potassium

4. Water needs vary greatly depending on:

    a. the food a person eats
    b. the environmental temperature and humidity
    c. the person's gender
    d. a and b
    e. b and c

5. The body's proteins and some of its minerals prevent changes in the acid-base balance of its fluids by serving as:

    a. ions
    b. electrolytes
    c. buffers
    d. solutes

6. Adult bone loss is referred to as:

    a. rickets
    b. osteomalacia
    c. osteodystrophy
    d. osteoporosis

7. Which of the following is(are) characteristics of osteoporosis?

    a. bones become porous
    b. bones become fragile
    c. bones bend
    d. a and b
    e. b and c

8   Which of the following absorbs the greatest amount of calcium?

    a. infants
    b. pregnant women
    c. adolescents
    d. older adults

9. Which of the following is the best source of calcium?

    a. butter
    b. cream
    c. cream cheese
    d. yogurt

10. The minimum sodium requirement set for U.S. adults is _____ milligrams.

    a. 300
    b. 500
    c. 2400
    d. 3200

11. Processed and fast foods are the source of almost _____ percent of the salt in most people's diets.

    a. 15
    b. 35
    c. 52
    d. 75

12. The most productive step to take to control salt intake is to:

    a. stop using instant foods
    b. discontinue the use of milk products
    c. limit intake of processed and fast foods
    d. control use of the salt shaker

13. Which of the following can cause potassium depletion?

    a. use of diuretics that cause potassium loss
    b. severe diarrhea
    c. excessive use of potassium chloride
    d. a and b
    e. b and c

14. Which of the following is part of the hydrochloric acid that maintains the strong acidity of the stomach?

    a. chloride
    b. sulfur
    c. magnesium
    d. potassium

15. Foods rich in magnesium are:

    a. slightly processed
    b. unprocessed
    c. highly processed
    d. a and c
    e. a and b

16. Which of the following is *not* a completely dependable source of iodine?

    a. seafood
    b. sea salt
    c. iodized salt
    d. plants grown in iodine-rich soil

17. All of the following are symptoms of iron-deficiency *except*:

    a. tiredness
    b. impaired concentration
    c. intolerance to heat
    d. apathy

18. Which of the following is often responsible for low iron intakes in the western world?

    a. blood loss caused by parasitic infections of the digestive tract
    b. malnutrition which includes an inadequate iron intake
    c. vegetarians who design their own meal patterns
    d. displacement of nutrient-rich foods by foods high in sugar and fat

19. The usual source of fluoride is:

    a. drinking water
    b. cooking utensils
    c. fortified foods
    d. processed foods

Application Level Items:

20. Which of the following determines whether calcium is withdrawn from or deposited to the skeleton?

    a. hormones that are sensitive to blood levels of calcium
    b. the amount of calcium consumed in the diet
    c. the amount of calcium deposited in bones during peak bone mass
    d. a and b
    e. b and c

21. Why is the intake recommendation for calcium set at 1300 milligrams/day for adolescents?

    a. because the skeleton begins to lose bone density during that age
    b. because people develop their peak bone mass during this time
    c. because a high calcium intake is thought to maximize bone density during the growing years
    d. a and b
    e. b and c

22. Which of the following provides the best choices for high calcium food selections?

    a. ice milk, cottage cheese, butter, and cream
    b. milk, buttermilk, cheese, and yogurt
    c. cream cheese, chocolate milk, and frozen yogurt
    d. sardines, spinach, kale, and swiss chard

23. How much sodium is consumed by someone who eats five grams of salt?

    a. 1000 mg
    b. 1500 mg
    c. 2000 mg
    d. 2500 mg

24. An increase in iodine intake in the United States has resulted from:

    a. dough conditioners used in the baking industry
    b. milk produced in dairies that feed cows iodine-containing medications
    c. the increased consumption of fast foods and convenience items
    d. a and b
    e. a and c

25. To improve the absorption of iron from an iron supplement you would:

    a. take the supplement with orange juice
    b. take the supplement with tea
    c. consume a small amount of meat along with the supplement
    d. a and b
    e. a and c

ANSWERS

SUMMING UP

(1) 60; (2) satiety; (3) thirst; (4) kidneys; (5) weight; (6) water; (7) balance; (8) transportation; (9) temperature; (10) calorie; (11) 2-3; (12) magnesium, (13) sodium; (14) cells; (15) outsides; (16) minerals; (17) electrolytes; (18) fluid; (19) acid-base; (20) bases; (21) abundant; (22) tooth; (23) nerve; (24) osteoporosis; (25) 1,300; (26) outside; (27) 40; (28) acid-base; (29) moderation; (30) diuretics; (31) sulfur; (32) chloride; (33) thyroxine; (34) iron; (35) myoglobin; (36) enzymes; (37) teeth

CHAPTER GLOSSARY

Matching Exercise 1: (1) e; (2) j; (3) g; (4) b; (5) r; (6) d; (7) o; (8) k; (9) a; (10) q; (11) m; (12) h; (13) l; (14) f; (15) p; (16) i; (17) c; (18) n
Matching Exercise 2: (1) f; (2) l; (3) h; (4) p; (5) b; (6) n; (7) e; (8) j; (9) o; (10) c; (11) m; (12) i; (13) g; (14) a; (15) k; (16) d; (17) r; (18) q

EXERCISES

Chapter Study Questions:

1. Hard water has high concentrations of calcium and magnesium, while soft water's principal mineral is sodium. Soft water adds appreciable amounts of sodium to the diet and may aggravate hypertension and heart disease.

2. Because absorption of calcium varies not only with age, but also with a person's vitamin D status and the calcium content of the diet.

3. Because people develop their peak bone mass, which is the highest attainable bone density for an individual, during childhood and young adulthood. Calcium absorption declines with age.

4. Diuretics are medications which cause increased water excretion and dehydration which leads to potassium loss from inside cells. It is especially dangerous because potassium loss from brain cells makes the victim unaware of the need for water. Potassium-rich foods are necessary to compensate for the losses.

5. Pica is a craving for non-food substances, such as ice, clay or paste, and is associated with iron-deficiency.

Short Answer Questions:

1. (a) calcium; (b) chloride; (c) magnesium; (d) phosphorus; (e) potassium; (f) sodium; (g) sulfur

2. (a) calcium; (b) magnesium; (c) sodium

3. (a) regulates transport of ions across cell membranes and is important in nerve transmission; (b) helps maintain normal blood pressure; (c) is essential for muscle contraction and maintenance of heartbeat; (d) plays a role in clotting of blood; (e) allows secretion of hormones, digestive enzymes, and neurotransmitters; (f) activates cellular enzymes that regulate many processes.

4. (a) overly strict use of low sodium diets; (b) vomiting; (c) diarrhea; (d) heaving sweating

5. (a) learn to control use of the salt shaker; (b) limit intake of processed and fast foods

6. (a) inadequate intake; (b) vomiting; (c) diarrhea; (d) alcoholism; (e) protein malnutrition

7. (a) seafood; (b) iodized salt

8. (a) tannins of tea and coffee; (b) calcium and phosphorus in milk; (c) phytates in whole grain cereals

Problem-Solving:

Decrease the amount of salt; substitute 1/4 cup oil for the 1/3 cup lard; use fresh or frozen green peas rather than canned green peas; substitute 2 tbsp. margarine for the 1/4 cup butter; delete the poultry seasoning; use unsalted and fat-free chicken broth; substitute skim milk for the cream.

Controversy Questions:

1. Trabecular bone is the web-like structure composed of calcium-containing crystals inside a bone's solid outer shell; it provides strength and acts as a calcium storage bank; cortical bone is the dense, ivory-like bone that forms the exterior shell of a bone and the shaft of a long bone; it provides a sturdy outer wall.

2. Poor nutrition involving calcium and vitamin D; estrogen deficiency in women; lack of physical activity; being underweight; use of alcohol and tobacco; and excess protein, sodium, caffeine, and soft drinks and inadequate vitamin K.

3. It is thought that genetic inheritance influences the maximum bone mass possible during growth and the extent of a woman's bone loss during menopause.

4. Weight-bearing exercises such as calisthenics, dancing, jogging, vigorous walking or weight training

5. Because divided doses can improve a day's total absorption up to 20 percent

STUDY AIDS

Major Minerals

Name	*Chief Functions*	*Deficiency Disease Name*	*Food Sources*
Calcium	makes up bone and **teeth** structure normal muscle contraction nerve functioning blood **clotting** immune defenses	**osteoporosis**	milk small **fish** with bones tofu greens legumes
Magnesium	**bone** mineralization building of protein normal muscle contraction transmission of nerve **impulses** maintenance of **teeth**		nuts **legumes** whole grains dark green **vegetables** seafoods **chocolate** cocoa
Sodium	maintains normal fluid balance maintains normal **acid-base** balance		salt **processed** foods **soy** sauce

Trace Minerals

Name	Chief Functions	Deficiency Disease Name	Food Sources
Iron	part of the protein **hemoglobin** part of the protein myoglobin necessary for utilization of **energy** in the body	**anemia**	**red** meats **fish** poultry shellfish eggs legumes **dried** fruits
Iodine	component of thyroid hormone **thyroxine**	**goiter** **cretinism**	**seafood** **iodized** salt bread
Zinc	part of insulin and many **enzymes** normal **fetal** development		**protein**-containing foods

SAMPLE TEST ITEMS

1. c (p. 266)	9. d (p. 298)	17. c (p. 287)
2. d (p. 269)	10. b (p. 281)	18. d (p. 288)
3. a (p. 270)	11. d (p. 282)	19. a (p. 293)
4. d (p. 269)	12. c (p. 282)	20. a (p. 276)
5. c (p. 275)	13. d (p. 284)	21. e (p. 277)
6. d (p. 276)	14. a (p. 285)	22. b (p. 298)
7. d (p. 276)	15. e (p. 279)	23. c (p. 280)
8. a (p. 277)	16. b (p. 286)	24. e (p. 286)
		25. e (p. 289)

CHAPTER 9

Energy Balance and Healthy Body Weight

CHAPTER OBJECTIVES

After completing this chapter, you should be able to:

1. List and define the three components of the body's energy budget.

2. Identify and explain the factors that affect the basal metabolic rate.

3. Estimate his or her individual total energy expenditure.

4. Discuss the problems of too much or too little body fat.

5. Describe health risks associated with central obesity and those groups most likely to be affected.

6. Discuss the role of BMI in evaluating obesity.

7. Evaluate the methods used for estimating body fatness.

8. Summarize the theories that attempt to explain the mystery of obesity.

9. Explain what happens during moderate weight loss versus rapid weight loss.

10. Summarize the recommended strategies to promote weight control.

11. Define and describe eating disorders and explain the physical harm that occurs as a result of these behaviors (Controversy 9).

KEY CONCEPTS

✓ Deficient body fatness threatens survival during a famine or in wasting diseases.

✓ Obesity has been named a chronic disease. Central obesity may be more hazardous to health than other forms of obesity. National guidelines for evaluating risks to health from obesity define obesity as a BMI of 30 or above. Overfatness presents social and economic handicaps as well as physical ills. Judging people by their body weight is a form of prejudice in our society.

✓ The "energy in" side of the body's energy budget is measured in calories taken in each day in the form of foods and beverages. The number of calories in foods and beverages can be obtained from published tables or computer diet analysis programs.

✓ Two major components of the "energy out" side of the body's energy budget are basal metabolism and voluntary activities. A third minor component of energy expenditures is the thermic effect of food.

✓ To estimate the energy spent on basal metabolism, use the factor 1.0 calorie (for men) or 0.9 calorie (for women) per kilogram of body weight per hour for a 24 hour period. Then add a percentage of this amount to account for daily expenditures in muscular activity.

✓ The body mass index mathematically correlates heights and weights with risks to health. It is especially useful for evaluating health risks of obesity but fails to measure body composition or fat distribution.

✓ A clinician can determine the percentage of fat in a person's body by measuring fatfolds, body density, or other parameters. Distribution of fat can be estimated by radiographic techniques and central adiposity by measuring waist circumference.

✓ No single body composition suits everyone; needs vary by gender, lifestyle, and stage of life.

✓ Food intake is regulated by hunger, appetite, satiation, and satiety. Discoveries of neural and hormonal regulators of eating behaviors may lead to new effective pharmacological treatments of obesity. Some foods may confer greater satiety than others.

✓ Inside-the-body causes of obesity include a person's genetic inheritance and its expression in terms of the handling of energy by the tissues. Energy-wasting proteins help to maintain normal body weight when food energy intake exceeds need. Leptin, a peptide hormone secreted by the adipose tissue, suppresses the appetite.

✓ Studies of human behavior identify stimuli that lead to eating and exercise habits. Physical inactivity is clearly linked with overfatness. Obesity treatment involves diet, exercise, and behavior modification.

✓ When energy balance is negative, glycogen returns glucose to the body. When glycogen runs out, body protein is called upon for glucose. Fat also supplies fuel as fatty acids. If glucose runs out, fat supplies fuel as ketone bodies, but ketosis can be dangerous. Both fasts and low-carbohydrate diets are ill-advised. People who successfully lose weight and keep it off eat abundant carbohydrates.

✓ When energy balance is positive, carbohydrate is converted to glycogen or fat, protein is converted to fat, and food fat is stored as fat. Alcohol delivers calories and encourages fat storage.

✓ To achieve and maintain a healthy body weight, set realistic goals, keep records, and expect to progress slowly. Make the diet adequate, limit fat and calories, reduce alcohol, and eat regularly.

✓ Weight gain requires a diet of calorie-dense foods, eaten frequently throughout the day. Physical activity builds lean tissue.

✓ Surgery and drugs to reduce body fatness may be risky, but severe obesity may be more risky still. Herbs and other gimmicks are useless, and some are dangerous.

✓ People who succeed at maintaining lost weight keep to their eating routines, keep exercising, and keep track of calorie and fat intakes and body weight. The more traits related to positive self-image and self-efficiency a person possesses or cultivates, the more likely that person will succeed.

SUMMING UP

Both deficient and (1) _____ body fat present health risks. For example,

underweight increases the risk for any person fighting a (2) _____ disease, while

overfatness can precipitate (3) _____ and thus increase the risk of stroke. Being

fat also triples a person's risk of developing (4) _____.

(5) _____ obesity may be more hazardous to health than other forms of obesity.

The "energy in" side of the body's energy budget is measured in (6) _____

taken in each day in the form of foods and beverages. Calories in foods and beverages can be

obtained from published tables or (7) _____ programs. The body spends energy

in two major ways: to fuel its (8) _____ metabolism and to fuel its

(9) _____ activities.

The (10) _____, which defines average relative weight for height,

usually correlates with body fatness and degree of disease risk. A clinician can determine the

percentage of fat in a person's body by measuring fatfolds, body (11) _____ , or

other parameters. Distribution of fat can be estimated by radiographic techniques and central

adiposity by measuring (12) _____ circumference.

Two schools of thought attempt to explain the development of obesity, with one attributing it to internal factors and the other to (13) _____ factors. One long-popular theory suggests that the body chooses a weight it wants to maintain and defends that weight and is referred to as the (14) _____ theory. A different line of research contends that obesity is determined by behavioral responses to environmental stimuli, which forms the basis for the (15) _____ cue theory. Physical (16) _____ is clearly linked with overfatness.

Researchers are interested in why people eat when and what they eat, and especially why some people overeat, and this has lead to investigations of hunger, (17) _____, and satiety. Hunger is the (18) _____ need to eat, while appetite is (19) _____. The perception of (20) _____ that lingers in the hours after a meal is called satiety. (21)_____ is a hormone produced by the adipose tissue that is directly linked to both appetite and body fatness.

Changes in body weight can reflect shifts in body (22) _____ content, in bone minerals, or in (23)_____ tissues such as muscles. The type of (24) _____ gained or lost depends on how the person goes about gaining or losing it. With prolonged fasting or carbohydrate deprivation, the body adapts by converting (25) _____ into compounds that the nervous system can adapt to use and this condition is called (26) _____.

Many different approaches to weight loss are used including fasting and low (27) _____ diets which are ill-advised. People who successfully lose weight and keep it off eat diets high in (28) _____ and low in fat.

CHAPTER GLOSSARY

Matching Exercise 1:

_____ 1. leptin

_____ 2. arousal

_____ 3. thermogenesis

_____ 4. wasting

_____ 5. appetite

_____ 6. thermic effect of food

_____ 7. satiety

_____ 8. set-point theory

_____ 9. adipose tissue

_____ 10. ketone bodies

_____ 11. body composition

_____ 12. gastroplasty

_____ 13. lipoprotein lipase

_____ 14. hunger

_____ 15. bioelectrical impedance

a. the body's speeded-up metabolism in response to having eaten a meal

b. acidic compounds derived from fat and certain amino acids

c. a technique to measure body fatness by measuring the body's degree of electrical conductivity

d. an appetite-suppressing hormone produced in the fat cells that conveys information about body fatness to the brain

e. the theory that the body tends to maintain a certain weight by means of its own internal controls

f. an enzyme mounted on the surfaces of fat cells that splits triglycerides in the blood into fatty acids and glycerol to be absorbed into the cells for reassembly and storage

g. the generation and release of body heat associated with the breakdown of body fuels

h. the body's fat tissue, consisting of masses of fat-storing cells and blood vessels to nourish them

i. surgery that partitions the stomach by stapling off a "pouch" or otherwise modifying the stomach, thereby reducing total food intake

j. the psychological desire to eat; a learned motivation and a positive sensation that accompanies the sight, smell, or thought of appealing foods

k. the proportions of muscle, bone, fat, and other tissue that make up a person's total body weight

l. heightened activity of certain brain centers associated with attention, excitement, and anxiety

m. the physiological need to eat, experienced as a drive for obtaining food; an unpleasant sensation that demands relief

n. the progressive, relentless loss of the body's tissues that accompanies certain diseases and shortens survival time

o. the perception of fullness that lingers in the hours after a meal and inhibits eating until the next mealtime

Matching Exercise 2:

_____ 1. subcutaneous fat

_____ 2. self-efficacy

_____ 3. visceral fat

_____ 4. endorphins

_____ 5. cellulite

_____ 6. DEXA

_____ 7. basal metabolic rate

_____ 8. basal metabolism

_____ 9. voluntary activities

_____ 10. underwater weighing

_____ 11. obesity

_____ 12. central obesity

_____ 13. fatfold test

_____ 14. weight cycling

_____ 15. body mass index

_____ 16. gastric bypass

a. a person's belief in his or her ability to succeed in an undertaking

b. the rate at which the body uses energy to support its basal metabolism

c. excess fat in the abdomen and around the trunk

d. an indicator of obesity, calculated by dividing the weight of a person by the square of the person's height

e. a term popularly used to describe dimpled fat tissue on the thighs and buttocks; not recognized in science

f. measurement of the thickness of a fold of skin on the back of the arm (over the triceps muscle), below the shoulder blade (subscapular), or in other places, using a caliper

g. fat stored directly under the skin

h. a measure of density and volume used to determine body fat content

i. fat stored within the abdominal cavity in association with the internal abdominal organs

j. overfatness, with adverse health effects

k. the sum total of all the involuntary activities that are necessary to sustain life, including respiration, circulation, and new tissue synthesis, but excluding digestion and voluntary activities

l. repeated rounds of weight loss and subsequent regain, with reduced ability to lose weight with each attempt

m. compounds of the brain whose actions mimic those of opiate drugs in reducing pain and producing pleasure

n. intentional activities conducted by voluntary muscles

o. a noninvasive method of determing total body fat, fat distribution and bone density

p. surgery that reroutes food from the stomach to the lower part of the small intestine

EXERCISES

Answer these chapter study questions:

1. What are risks associated with being underweight?

2. Why is body weight an unsatisfactory indicator of health or risk status?

3. Identify appropriate strategies for weight gain.

4. Describe diet-related changes that most often lead to successful weight change and maintenance.

5.   Describe how exercise can increase the BMR.

Complete these short answer questions:

1.   Obese adults are at excess risk for these conditions:

a.   i.
b.   j.
c.   k.
d.   l.
e.   m.
f.   n.
g.   o.
h.   p.

2.   Two major components of the "energy out" side of the body's energy budget are:

a.
b.

3.   Body mass index is unsuitable for use with:

a.
b.
c.

4.   Basal metabolism includes:

a.   d.
b.   e.
c.   f.

5.   Food intake is regulated by:

a.
b.
c.
d.

6. The best treatment for most overweight people boils down to control in three areas:

    a.
    b.
    c.

7. Changes in body weight may reflect shifts in any of the following materials:

    a.
    b.
    c.
    d.

8. The three kinds of energy nutrients are stored in the body in two forms, including _____ and _____ .

9. Physiological hazards that accompany low-carbohydrate diets include:

    a.
    b.
    c.
    d.

10. In late food deprivation, _____ bodies help feed the nervous system and so help spare tissue protein.

Solve these problems:

1. Calculate the energy needs for a 110 pound female who works as a teacher.

2. Using the Exchange System, calculate the number of calories provided by the following meal:

Food Item	*Amount*	*Number of Calories*
Boiled egg	1	_____
Whole wheat toast	1 slice	_____
Margarine	2 teaspoons	_____
Grapefruit	1/2	_____
Skim milk	1 cup	_____
		TOTAL: _____

3. Calculate the grams of carbohydrate, protein, and fat which should be supplied in a 1000 calorie diet, using the distribution of 50% carbohydrate, 25% protein, and 25% fat.

Solve these controversy questions:

1. What are the three associated medical problems that form the female athlete triad?

2. What are three characteristics specific to anorexia nervosa?

3. What two issues and behaviors must be addressed in the treatment of anorexia nervosa?

4. Differentiate between the two types of bulimia nervosa?

5. What are the two primary goals of treatment for bulimia nervosa?

STUDY AID

Identify whether the following factors are associated with a higher or lower *Basal Metabolic Rate (BMR)* by placing an X in the appropriate space.

	Factor	*Higher BMR*	*Lower BMR*
a.	Youth	____	____
b.	Being tall and thin	____	____
c.	Fasting/Starvation	____	____
d.	Heat	____	____
e.	Malnutrition	____	____
f.	Stress hormones	____	____
g.	Pregnant women	____	____
h.	Fever	____	____
i.	Thyroxine	____	____

SAMPLE TEST ITEMS

Comprehension Level Items:

1. Health risks associated with excessive body fat include all of the following *except:*

    a. increased risk of developing hypertension
    b. increased risk for developing ulcers
    c. increased risk for heart disease
    d. increased risk for developing diabetes

2. Which of the following groups is *least* likely to carry more intraabdominal fat?

    a. men
    b. women in their reproductive years
    c. women past menopause
    d. smokers

3. Obesity is officially defined as a body mass index of 30 or higher.

    a. true
    b. false

4. The external cue theory of obesity suggests that:

    a. people eat in response to internal factors
    b. people eat in response to factors such as hunger
    c. environmental influences override internal regulatory systems
    d. the body tends to maintain a certain weight by means of external controls

5. A man of normal weight may have, on the average, _____ percent of the body weight as fat.

    a. 5-10
    b. 10-15
    c. 12-20
    d. 20-30

6. BMI values are most valuable for evaluating degrees of obesity and are less useful for evaluating nonobese people's body fatness.

    a. true
    b. false

7. Central obesity correlates with an increased incidence of:

    a. diabetes
    b. kidney disease
    c. stroke
    d. a and b
    e. a and c

153

8. The theory that the body tends to maintain a certain weight by means of its own internal controls is called the _____ theory.

    a. enzyme
    b. set-point
    c. thermogenesis
    d. fat cell

9. Which of the following helps to feed the brain during times when too little carbohydrate is available?

    a. lipoprotein lipase
    b. brown fat
    c. ketone bodies
    d. leptin

10. A diet moderately restricted in calories has been observed to promote a greater rate of weight loss, a faster rate of fat loss, and retention of more lean tissue than a severely restricted fast.

    a. true
    b. false

11. Which of the following largely determines whether weight is gained as body fat or as lean tissue?

    a. the number of calories consumed
    b. the amount of fat consumed
    c. the person's current body composition
    d. exercise

12. Hunger makes itself known roughly _____ hours after eating.

    a. 2 - 4
    b. 4 - 6
    c. 8 - 12
    d. 12 - 14

13. Ketone bodies are:

    a. acidic compounds
    b. derived from fat
    c. normally present in the blood
    d. a and b
    e. b and c

14. Which of the following directly controls basal metabolism?

    a. epinephrine
    b. insulin
    c. thyroxine
    d. lipase

15. Which of the following statements is ***not*** true?

    a. any food can make you fat if you eat enough of it
    b. alcohol both delivers calories and encourages fat accumulation
    c. fat from food, as opposed to carbohydrate or protein, is especially easy for the body to store as fat tissue
    d. protein, once converted to fat, can later be recovered as amino acids

16. Diet strategies for weight loss should include all of the following ***except***:

    a. skipping meals
    b. eating controlled portions
    c. eating meals at a leisurely pace
    d. eating before being very hungry

17. Fatfold measurements provide an accurate estimate of total body fat and a fair assessment of the fat's location.

    a. true
    b. false

18. Which of the following is the first element in implementing a behavior modification program?

    a. reward yourself personally and immediately
    b. strengthen cues to appropriate behaviors
    c. eliminate inappropriate eating cues
    d. arrange negative consequences for negative behaviors

19. All of the following are considered to be part of basal metabolism ***except:***

    a. beating of the heart
    b. inhaling and exhaling of air
    c. maintenance of body temperature
    d. sitting and walking

Application Level Items:

20. Kathy weighs 140 pounds and has a body mass index of 28. Based on this information you would classify her as:

    a. underweight
    b. normal weight
    c. overweight
    d. obese

21. John has a body mass index of 31, therefore, you would classify him as:

    a. underweight
    b. normal weight
    c. overweight
    d. obese

22. Susie is underweight and wishes to gain weight. Which of the following should she do?

    a. exercise
    b. eat only three meals a day
    c. eat a high-calorie diet
    d. a and b
    e. a and c

23. Emily has been overweight most of her life and she has been on almost every type of diet possible. Although she loses weight initially on reducing diets, she subsequently returns to her original weight. Which of the following theories could explain Emily's problem with being overweight?

    a. fat cell theory
    b. set-point theory
    c. external cue theory
    d. enzyme theory

24. Sarah is bragging about losing 10 pounds in one week on a weight loss program. What would you tell Sarah?

    a. it's great that you have lost that much weight so fast
    b. you need to slow down your rate of weight loss
    c. the weight loss probably represents changes in body fluid content
    d. your change in weight probably reflects a loss of body fat

25. Karen is interested in speeding up her basal metabolic rate to promote fat loss. You would advise her to:

    a. eat smaller meals more frequently throughout the day
    b. participate in endurance and strength-building exercise daily
    c. fast at least one day each week
    d. follow a low carbohydrate diet

ANSWERS

SUMMING UP

(1) excessive; (2) wasting; (3) hypertension; (4) diabetes; (5) central; (6) calories;
(7) computer diet analysis; (8) basal; (9) voluntary; (10) body mass index; (11) density;
(12) waist; (13) external; (14) set-point; (15) external; (16) inactivity; (17) appetite;
(18) physiological; (19) psychological; (20) fullness; (21) leptin; (22) fluid; (23) lean;
(24) tissue; (25) fat; (26) ketosis; (27) carbohydrate; (28) carbohydrates

CHAPTER GLOSSARY

Matching Exercise 1: (1) d; (2) l; (3) g; (4) n; (5) j; (6) a; (7) o; (8) e; (9) h; (10) b; (11) k;
(12) i; (13) f; (14) m; (15) c
Matching Exercise 2: (1) g; (2) a; (3) i; (4) m; (5) e; (6) o; (7) b; (8) k; (9) n; (10) h; (11) j;
(12) c; (13) f; (14) l; (15) d; (16) p

EXERCISES

Chapter Study Questions:

1. Overly thin people are at a disadvantage in the hospital where they may have to refrain from eating food for days at a time so that they can undergo tests or surgery and their nutrient status can easily deteriorate. Underweight also increases the risk for any person fighting a wasting disease such as cancer.

2. Because body weight says little about composition. For example, a healthy person may have dense bones and muscles and seem overweight on a scale, while a person whose scale weight seems reasonable may have too much body fat for health.

3. Participate in physical activity; increase calories and learn to eat nutritious, calorie-dense foods; and eat more frequently.

4. Keep records of food intake and exercise habits; set goals; plan a diet with foods you like; pay attention to portions; plan high-fiber and carbohydrate foods into the diet; eat regularly; include breakfast; cut down on or eliminate alcohol.

5. Exercise helps body composition change toward the lean. Lean tissue is more metabolically active than fat tissue, so the basal energy output picks up the pace as well.

Short Answer Questions:

1. (a) hypertension; (b) diabetes; (c) cardiovascular disease; (d) respiratory problems; (e) liver malfunction; (f) high blood lipids; (g) sleep apnea; (h) some cancers; (i) varicose veins; (j) gout; (k) gallbladder disease; (l) complications in pregnancy and surgery; (m) high accident rate; (n) flat feet, (o) abdominal hernias; (p) arthritis

2. (a) basal metabolism; (b) voluntary activities

3. (a) athletes; (b) adults over 65; (c) pregnant and lactating women

4. (a) circulation; (b) respiration; (c) temperature maintenance; (d) hormone secretion; (e) nerve activity; (f) new tissue synthesis

5. (a) hunger; (b) appetite; (c) satiation; (d) satiety

6. (a) diet; (b) physical activity; (c) behavior modification

7. (a) fluid content; (b) bone minerals; (c) lean tissue; (d) contents of the bladder or digestive tract

8. glycogen; fat

9. (a) high blood cholesterol and gallbladder disease; (b) hypoglycemia; (c) lack of needed nutrients and phytochemicals; (d) digestive track ailments

10. ketone

Problem-Solving:

1. (a) change pounds to kilograms: 110 pounds divided by 2.2. pounds = 50 kilograms; (b) multiply weight in kilograms by the BMR factor: 50 kilograms x 0.9 calories per kilogram per hour = 45 calories per hour; (c) multiply the calories used in one hour by the hours in a day: 45 calories per hour x 24 hours per day = 1080 calories per day; (d) multiply BMR calories per day by 40-60%: 1080 calories per day x 40 percent = 432 calories per day for activities; 60 percent = 648 calories; (e) total BMR calories and activities calories: 1080 calories per day + 432 calories per day = 1512 calories per day; 1080 + 648 = 1728 calories per day; (f) total energy equals between 1512 and 1728 calories per day

2.

Food Item	Amount	Number of Calories
Boiled egg	1	75
Whole wheat toast	1 slice	80
Margarine	2 teaspoons	90
Grapefruit	1/2	60
Skim milk	1 cup	90
	TOTAL:	395

3. (a) 50% carbohydrate x 1000 calories = 500 carbohydrate calories divided by 4 calories per gram = 125 grams carbohydrate; (b) 25% protein x 1000 calories = 250 protein calories divided by 4 calories per gram = 63 grams protein; (c) 25% fat x 1000 calories = 250 fat calories divided by 9 calories per gram = 28 grams fat

Controversy Questions:

1. Disordered eating, amenorrhea, and osteoporosis

2. A refusal to maintain a minimally normal body weight, self-starvation to the extreme, and a disturbed perception of body weight and shape

3. Those relating to food and weight and those involving relationships with oneself and others

4. The purging type is where the person regularly engages in self-induced vomiting or the misuse of laxatives, diuretics or enemas; the non-purging type is when the person uses other inappropriate compensatory behaviors, such as fasting or excessive exercise, but not vomiting, laxatives, diuretics or enemas.

5. Steady maintenance of weight and prevention of relapse into cyclic gains and losses.

STUDY AID

	Factor	Higher BMR	Lower BMR
a.	Youth	x	
b.	Being tall and thin	x	
c.	Fasting/Starvation		x
d.	Heat	x	
e.	Malnutrition		x
f.	Stress hormones	x	
g.	Pregnant women	x	
h.	Fever	x	
i.	Thyroxine	x	

SAMPLE TEST ITEMS

1. b (p. 313)
2. b (p. 313)
3. a (p. 313)
4. c (p. 326-327)
5. c (p. 321)
6. a (p. 318)
7. e (p. 313)
8. b (p. 324)

9. c (p. 333)
10. a (p. 333)
11. d (p. 339)
12. b (p. 322)
13. d (p. 333)
14. c (p. 316)
15. d (p. 336)
16. a (p. 337-339)

17. a (p. 320)
18. c (p. 345)
19. d (p. 316)
20. c (p. 312)
21. d (p. 312)
22. e (p. 339-340)
23. b (p. 324)
24. c (p. 331-332)
25. b (p. 316-317)

CHAPTER 10

Nutrients, Physical Activity, and the Body's Responses

CHAPTER OBJECTIVES

After completing this chapter, you should be able to:

1. Explain the benefits of and guidelines for regular physical activity for the body.

2. Describe the components of fitness and how muscles respond to physical activity.

3. Summarize how the body adjusts its fuel mix to respond to physical activity of varying intensity levels and duration.

4. Explain the concepts of carbohydrate loading.

5. Discuss the roles vitamins and minerals play in physical performance and indicate whether supplements are necessary to support the needs of active people.

6. Describe the importance of fluids and temperature regulation in physical activity and the best way to stay hydrated before and during exercise.

7. Describe the characteristics of the most appropriate diet for athletes.

8. List the risks of taking *"ergogenic"* aids and steroids to enhance physical performance. (Controversy 10)

KEY CONCEPTS

✓ Physical activity and fitness benefit people's physical and psychological well-being and improve their resistance to disease. Physical activity to improve physical fitness eases the tasks of daily living and offers additional personal benefits.

✓ The components of fitness are flexibility, muscle strength, muscle endurance, and cardiorespiratory endurance. To build fitness, a person must engage in physical activity. Muscles adapt to activities they are called upon to perform.

✓ Weight training offers health and fitness benefits to adults. Weight training reduces the risk of cardiovascular disease, improves older adults' physical mobility, and helps maximize and maintain bone mass.

✓ Cardiorespiratory endurance training enhances the ability of the heart and lungs to deliver oxygen to the muscles. With cardiorespiratory endurance training, the heart becomes stronger, breathing becomes more efficient, and the health of the entire body improves.

✓ Glucose is supplied by dietary carbohydrate or made by the liver. It is stored in both liver and muscle tissue as glycogen. Total glycogen stores affect an athlete's endurance.

✓ The more intense an activity, the more glucose it demands. During anaerobic metabolism, the body spends glucose rapidly and accumulates lactic acid.

✓ Physical activity of long duration places demands on the body's glycogen stores. Carbohydrate ingested before and during long-duration activity may help to forestall hypoglycemia and fatigue. Carbohydrate loading is a regimen of physical activity and diet that enables an athlete's muscles to store larger-than-normal amounts of glycogen to extend endurance. After strenuous training, eating foods with a high glycemic index may help restore glycogen most rapidly.

✓ Highly trained muscles use less glucose and more fat than do untrained muscles to perform the same work, so their glycogen lasts longer.

✓ Athletes who eat high-fat diets may burn more fat during endurance activity, but the risks to health outweigh any possible performance benefits. The intensity and duration of activity, as well as the degree of training, affect fat use.

✓ Physical activity stimulates muscle cells to break down and synthesize protein, resulting in muscle adaptation to activity. Athletes use protein both for building muscle tissue and for energy. Diet, intensity and duration of activity, and training affect protein use during activity.

✓ Vitamins are essential for releasing the energy trapped in energy-yielding nutrients and for other functions that support physical activity. Active people can meet their vitamin needs if they eat enough nutrient-dense foods to meet their energy needs.

✓ Moderate physical activity strengthens the bones, but young women athletes who train strenuously, become amenorrheic, and practice abnormal eating behaviors are susceptible to stress fractures and osteoporosis.

✓ Iron-deficiency anemia impairs physical performance because iron is the blood's oxygen handler. Sports anemia is a harmless temporary adaptation to physical activity.

✓ The body adapts to compensate for sweat losses of electrolytes, but urinary potassium losses may persist. Athletes are advised to use foods, not supplements, to make up for those losses.

✓ Evaporation of sweat cools the body. Heat stroke can be a threat to physically active people in hot, humid weather. Hypothermia threatens those who exercise in the cold.

✓ Physically active people lose fluids and must replace them to avoid dehydration. Thirst indicates that water loss has already occurred.

✓ Water is the best drink for most physically active people, but endurance athletes need drinks that supply glucose as well as fluids.

✓ Caffeine-containing drinks within limits may not impair performance, but water and fruit juice are preferred. Alcohol use can impair performance in many ways and is not recommended.

SUMMING UP

Physical activity benefits people's physical and psychological well-being and improves their resistance to (1) _____. Fitness is composed of four components including flexibility, muscle (2) _____, (3) _____ endurance and cardiorespiratory endurance. Muscle cells and tissues respond to an (4) _____ of physical activity by gaining strength and size, a response called (5) _____. The kind of exercise that brings about cardiorespiratory endurance is (6) _____ activity. In contrast, (7) _____ enhances flexibility and weight training and calisthenics develop (8) _____ strength and endurance and prevent and manage several chronic diseases.

The stored glucose of muscle (9) _____ is a major fuel for physical activity. How long an exercising person's glycogen will last depends not only on diet but also partly on the (10) _____ of the activity. Glycogen depletion usually occurs after about (11)_____ _____ hours of vigorous exercise. Glucose use during physical activity depends not only on the intensity, but also on the (12) _____ of the activity. A person who continues to exercise moderately for longer than 20 minutes begins to use less glucose and more (13) _____ for fuel. One diet strategy useful for endurance

athletes is to eat a high (14) _____ diet on a day-to-day basis.

The vitamin trio of thiamin, (15) _____, and niacin play key roles in

(16) _____release. Scientists have concluded, however, that extra amounts of these

vitamins provide no (17) _____ advantage. Vitamin (18) _____ seems

to be the most important antioxidant related to physical activity. Endurance athletes, and female

athletes in particular, are prone to (19)_____ deficiency.

Endurance athletes can lose (20) _____ or more quarts of fluid in every

hour of activity and must hydrate before, and rehydrate (21) _____ and after

activity to replace it all. Plain, cool (22) _____ is the best fluid for most active

bodies.

Athletes need a diet composed mostly of (23) _____dense foods, the

kind that supply a maximum of vitamins and minerals for the energy they provide. A diet that is

(24)_____ in carbohydrate, low in (25) _____, and adequate in

(26) _____ ensures full glycogen stores. The (27) _____ meal

should be light, easy to (28) _____ and should contain fluids. In addition, it

should be finished at least (29) _____ hours before competition.

CHAPTER GLOSSARY

Matching Exercise 1:

_____ 1. chromium picolinate

_____ 2. heat stroke

_____ 3. carbohydrate loading

_____ 4. pregame meal

_____ 5. branched-chain amino acids

_____ 6. stress fracture

_____ 7. lactic acid

_____ 8. ergogenic

_____ 9. hypothermia

_____ 10. human growth hormone

_____ 11. amenorrhea

_____ 12. ornithine

a. a bone injury or break caused by the stress of exercise on the bone surface

b. a hormone produced by the brain's pituitary gland that regulates normal growth and development

c. a trace element supplement falsely promoted to increase lean body mass, enhance energy, and burn fat

d. a nonessential amino acid falsely promoted as enhancing the secretion of human growth hormone, the breakdown of fat, and the development of muscle

e. a regimen of moderate exercise, followed by eating a high carbohydrate diet, that enables muscles to temporarily store glycogen beyond their normal capacity

f. the term implies _"energy giving"_

g. an acute and life threatening reaction to heat buildup in the body

h. a below-normal body temperature

i. amino acids that, unlike the others, can provide energy directly to muscle tissue; leucine, isoleucine, and valine

j. the absence or cessation of menstruation

k. a meal eaten three to four hours before athletic competition

l. a product of the incomplete breakdown of glucose during anaerobic metabolism

Matching Exercise 2:

____ 1. overload

____ 2. stroke volume

____ 3. myoglobin

____ 4. training

____ 5. muscle endurance

____ 6. flexibility

____ 7. cardiorespiratory endurance

____ 8. weight training

____ 9. hypertrophy

____ 10. cardiac output

____ 11. aerobic

____ 12. anaerobic

____ 13. VO$_2$ max

____ 14. atrophy

a. the ability of a muscle to contract repeatedly within a given time without becoming exhausted

b. an increase in size (for example, of a muscle) in response to use

c. not requiring oxygen

d. the muscles' iron-containing protein that stores and releases oxygen in response to the muscles' energy needs

e. the ability to perform large muscle dynamic exercise of moderate to high intensity for prolonged periods

f. a decrease in size of a muscle because of disuse

g. an extra physical demand placed on the body

h. requiring oxygen

i. the amount of oxygenated blood ejected from the heart toward body tissues at each beat

j. the capacity of the joints to move through a full range of motion; the ability to bend and recover without injury

k. the volume of blood discharged by the heart each minute

l. regular practice of an activity, which leads to physical adaptations of the body, with improvements in flexibility, strength, or endurance

m. the maximum rate of oxygen consumption by an individual (measured at sea level)

n. the use of free weights or weight machines to provide resistance for developing muscle strength and endurance

EXERCISES

Answer these chapter study questions:

1. Why is vitamin E especially important to endurance athletes?

2. Discuss possible causes of iron-deficiency in athletes.

3. What is the purpose of carbohydrate loading? Describe the steps involved.

4. What are two routes of significant water loss from the body during exercise? Which is the greater loss?

5. What is the best fluid for most exercising bodies? Why?

Complete these short answer questions:

1. The four components of fitness are:

    a.
    b.
    c.
    d.

2. Benefits of weight training include:

    a.
    b.
    c.

3. Branched-chain amino acids include:

    a.
    b.
    c.

4. Cardiorespiratory endurance is characterized by:

    a.
    b.
    c.
    d.
    e.
    f.

5. Fours strategies which endurance athletes use to try to maintain their blood glucose concentrations as long as they can include:

    a.
    b.
    c.
    d.

6. Factors that affect fat use during physical activity include:

    a.
    b.
    c.

7. Sweat and urine losses of these three trace minerals accelerate during physical activity:

    a.
    b.
    c.

8. Factors that affect how much protein is used during physical activity include:

   a.
   b.
   c.

9. Precautions to prevent heat stroke include:

   a.
   b.
   c.

10. The pregame meal should be eaten _____ hours before athletic competition.

Solve these problems:

1. An athlete weighs 150 pounds prior to a workout and 145 pounds after a workout. How much fluid should be consumed in order to rehydrate the body?

2. Review the example pregame meal below, determine all of the foods and/or beverages which would not be recommended, and identify an appropriate substitute for each non-recommended item.

	Substitute
orange juice	_____
3 ounce hamburger patty	_____
bun	_____
potato chips	_____
raw carrot sticks	_____
frozen yogurt	_____

Solve these controversy questions:

1. Explain why large doses of amino acid supplements can be dangerous.

2. What are some of the possible adverse effects of caffeine consumption among athletes?

3. What is the most appropriate way for an athlete to use a specialty drink or bar?

4. Which group of athletes is most likely to use steroids? Why?

5. Why is carnitine supplementation not necessary for an athlete?

STUDY AIDS

For questions 1-5, match the activities, listed on the left, with the type of fitness they develop, listed on the right.

_____1. weight training

_____2. repetitive exercises like push-ups

_____3. stretches

_____4. swimming

_____5. fast bicycling

a. flexibility

b. muscle strength and endurance

c. cardiorespiratory endurance

For questions 6-10, match the vitamins and minerals, listed on the right, with their exercise-related functions, listed on the left.

_____6. energy-releasing reactions

_____7. protects against bone loss

_____8. collagen formation for joint and other tissue integrity

_____9. transport of oxygen in blood and in muscle tissue

_____10. defends cell membranes against oxidation damage

a. iron

b. thiamin

c. calcium

d. vitamin C

e. vitamin E

11. Use the following tables in your textbook as study aids: Table 10-1 on page 361; Table 10-4 on page 377.

SAMPLE TEST ITEMS

Comprehension Level Items:

1. The ability to bend and recover without injury is called:

   a. fitness
   b. flexibility
   c. strength
   d. endurance

2. People who regularly engage in just moderate physical activity live longer on average than those who are physically inactive.

    a. true
    b. false

3. The average resting pulse rate for adults is around _____ beats per minute.

    a. 20
    b. 50
    c. 70
    d. 90

4. Which of the following produce cardiorespiratory endurance?

    a. swimming
    b. slow walking
    c. basketball
    d. a and b
    e. a and c

5. Sports anemia:

    a. is the same as iron-deficiency anemia
    b. reflects a normal adaptation to physical activity
    c. hinders the ability to perform work
    d. requires iron supplementation

6. A water loss of _____ percent of body weight can reduce a person's capacity to do muscular work.

    a. 1 - 2
    b. 3 - 4
    c. 5 - 6
    d. 7 - 8

7. Plain, cool water is the optimal beverage for replacing fluids in those who exercise because it:

    a. rapidly leaves the digestive tract
    b. takes a long time to enter the tissues
    c. cools the body from the inside out
    d. a and b
    e. a and c

8. Which of following beverages is recommended for an athlete?

    a. iced tea
    b. beer
    c. coffee
    d. fruit juice

9. To postpone exhaustion, endurance athletes should:

    a. eat a high carbohydrate diet on a day-to-day basis
    b. take in some glucose during exercise
    c. avoid carbohydrate-rich foods following exercise
    d. a and b
    e. b and c

10. Which of the following is an effect of regular physical activity?

    a. decreased lean body tissue
    b. less bone density
    c. reduced HDL cholesterol
    d. reduced risk of cardiovascular disease

11 Cardiorespiratory endurance is characterized by:

    a. increased heart strength and stroke volume
    b. improved circulation
    c. increased blood pressure
    d. a and b
    e. b and c

12. The American College of Sports Medicine's guidelines recommend that people spend an accumulated minimum of 30 minutes in some sort of physical activity on most days of the week.

    a. true
    b. false

13. Glycogen depletion usually occurs after about _____ hour(s) of vigorous exercise.

    a. 1/2
    b. 1
    c. 1 ½
    d. 2

14. The best strategy for dealing with lactic acid build-up is to:

    a. relax the muscles at every opportunity during activity
    b. stop exercising completely
    c. slow down the rate of exercise
    d. exercise at one-half of your usual pace

15. For athletes who exercise for an hour or more, sports drinks offer some advantages over water.

    a. true
    b. false

16. After about _____ minutes of activity the blood fatty acid concentration rises and surpasses the normal resting concentration.

    a. 10
    b. 20
    c. 30
    d. 45

17. All of the following factors affect fat use in exercise *except:*

    a. amount of fat in the diet
    b. degree of training to perform the exercise
    c. intensity and duration of the exercise
    d. area of the body involved in the exercise

18. Which of the following directs protein synthesis in building muscle?

    a. protein
    b. nutrients
    c. physical activity
    d. amino acids

19. All of the following minerals are excreted in larger amounts when people are physically active than when they are sedentary *except:*

    a. magnesium
    b. calcium
    c. zinc
    d. chromium

Application Level Items:

20. How would you respond to an athlete who states that branched-chain amino acid supplements should be taken because the branched-chain amino acids can directly provide energy to muscle tissue?

    a. ordinary foods cannot provide enough branched-chain amino acids
    b. the body prefers isolated amino acids to the combinations found in food
    c. when amino acids are needed, the muscles have plenty on hand
    d. a and b
    e. b and c

21. A male athlete weighs 175 pounds before a race and 168 pounds after a race. How much fluid should he consume?

    a. 8 cups
    b. 10 cups
    c. 12 cups
    d. 14 cups

22. Approximately how many grams of fat would an athlete need to consume to ensure full glycogen and other nutrient stores and to meet energy needs if she consumes 2500 calories?

    a. 40 grams
    b. 56 grams
    c. 75 grams
    d. 180 grams

23. Which of the following foods would be most appropriate as part of a pregame meal?

    a. baked potato with chili and sour cream
    b. marinated vegetable salad with whole wheat crackers
    c. salami on rye bread with mayonnaise
    d. pasta with steamed vegetables served with French bread

24. Why are people who exercise in humid, hot weather more susceptible to heat stroke?

    a. because they cannot judge how hot they are getting
    b. because they do not sweat under such conditions
    c. because sweat does not evaporate well under such conditions
    d. a and b
    e. b and c

25. Fred wishes to increase his basal metabolic rate. Which of the following should Fred do?

    a. engage in intense, prolonged activity
    b. drink iced tea
    c. eat a high carbohydrate diet
    d. drink plenty of water

ANSWERS

SUMMING UP

(1) disease; (2) strength; (3) muscle; (4) overload; (5) hypertrophy; (6) aerobic; (7) stretching; (8) muscle; (9) glycogen; (10) intensity; (11) two; (12) duration; (13) fat; (14) carbohydrate; (15) riboflavin; (16) energy; (17) competitive; (18) E; (19) iron; (20) two; (21) during; (22) water; (23) nutrient, (24) high; (25) fat; (26) protein; (27) pregame; (28) digest; (29) 3-4

CHAPTER GLOSSARY

Matching Exercise 1: (1) c; (2) g; (3) e; (4) k; (5) i; (6) a; (7) l; (8) f; (9) h; (10) b; (11) j; (12) d

Matching Exercise 2: (1) g; (2) i; (3) d; (4) l; (5) a; (6) j; (7) e; (8) n; (9) b; (10) k; (11) h; (12) c; (13) m; (14) f

EXERCISES

Chapter Study Questions:

1. During prolonged, high-intensity physical activity, the muscles' consumption of oxygen increases tenfold or more, enhancing the production of damaging free radicals in the body. Vitamin E is a potent fat-soluble antioxidant that vigorously defends the cell membranes against oxidative damage.

2. Marginal iron intakes may contribute to iron-deficiency. In addition, some destruction of red blood cells occurs when body tissues, such as the soles of the feet, make high-impact contact with an unyielding surface, such as the ground. Other explanations relate to the loss of iron through sweat, increased iron demand by muscles, and small blood losses through the digestive tract.

3. It is a technique used to trick the muscles into storing extra glycogen before a competition. During the week prior to competition, the athlete tapers training and then eats a diet that is high in carbohydrates during the three days before competition.

4. Water is lost from the body via sweat, which increases during exercise in order to rid the body of its excess heat by evaporation. In addition, breathing costs water, exhaled as vapor. Sweat is the greater way in which water loss occurs during exercise.

5. Plain, cool water because it rapidly leaves the digestive tract to enter the tissues, where it is needed, and it cools the body from the inside out.

Short Answer Questions:

1. (a) flexibility; (b) muscle strength; (c) muscle endurance; (d) cardiorespiratory endurance

2. (a) reduces risk of cardiovascular disease; (b) improves older adults' physical mobility; (c) helps maximize and maintain bone mass

3. (a) leucine; (b) isoleucine; (c) valine

4. (a) increased cardiac output and oxygen delivery; (b) increased heart strength and stroke volume; (c) slowed resting pulse; (d) increased breathing efficiency; (e) improved circulation; (f) reduced blood pressure

5. (a) eating a high carbohydrate diet on a day-to-day basis; (b) taking in some glucose during the activity; (c) training the muscles to store as much glycogen as possible; (d) eating carbohydrate-rich foods following activity to boost storage of glycogen

6. (a) fat intake; (b) intensity and duration of the activity; (c) degree of training

7. (a) chromium; (b) zinc; (c) magnesium

8. (a) carbohydrate intake; (b) intensity and duration of the activity; (c) degree of training

9. (a) drinking enough fluid before and during the activity; (b) resting in the shade when tired; (c) wearing light-weight clothing that encourages evaporation

10. 3-4

Problem-Solving:

1. One pound of body weight equals roughly two cups of fluid; since 5 pounds of weight were lost, approximately 10 cups of fluid should be consumed.

2.
	Substitute
orange juice	
3 ounce hamburger patty	**lean chicken breast**
bun	
potato chips	**baked potato**
raw carrot sticks	**steamed green beans**
frozen yogurt	

Controversy Questions:

1. Amino acids compete for carriers, and an overdose of one can limit the availability of some other needed amino acids, setting up both a possible toxicity of the supplemented one and a deficiency of the others.

2. Adverse effects include stomach upset, nervousness, irritability, headaches, dehydration, and diarrhea; it can also raise blood pressure above normal, making the heart work harder to pump blood to the working muscles.

3. The most appropriate way for an athlete to use specialty drinks and bars is as a pregame meal or between-meal snack.

4. Professional athletes, for which monetary rewards for excellence are high, are most likely to use steroids.

5. Because carnitine is a nonessential nutrient that the body makes for itself, plus it is contained in meat and milk products.

STUDY AIDS

(1) b; (2) b; (3) a; (4) c; (5) c; (6) b; (7) c; (8) d; (9) a; (10) e

SAMPLE TEST ITEMS

1. b (p. 361)	9. d (p. 367)	17. d (p. 370)
2. a (p. 360)	10. d (p. 361)	18. c (p. 371)
3. c (p. 363)	11. d (p. 363)	19. b (p. 375)
4. e (p. 363)	12. a (p. 360)	20. c (p. 370-372)
5. b (p. 374-375)	13. d (p. 366)	21. d (p. 376)
6. a (p. 375)	14. a (p. 367)	22. b (p. 380)
7. e (p. 376)	15. a (p. 378)	23. d (p. 382)
8. d (p. 379)	16. b (p. 370)	24. c (p. 376)
		25. a (p. 370-371)

CHAPTER 11

Diet and Health

CHAPTER OBJECTIVES

After completing this chapter, you should be able to:

1.   Describe the role of nutrition in maintaining a healthy immune system.

2.   Define atherosclerosis and identify the risk factors for cardiovascular disease.

3.   Describe how hypertension develops and identify the risk factors associated with this disease.

4.   Discuss the strategies that can be used to reduce the risks of cardiovascular disease and hypertension.

5.   Describe the process by which a cancer develops and explain what is known about the effects of food constituents on cancer development.

6.   Give some examples of common nutrient-drug interactions. (Controversy 11)

KEY CONCEPTS

✓   Adequate nutrition is a key component in maintaining a healthy immune system to defend against infectious diseases. Medical nutrition therapy can improve the course of wasting diseases. Both excessive and deficient nutrients can harm the immune system.

✓   The same diet and lifestyle risk factors may contribute to several degenerative diseases. A person's family history can reveal strategies for disease prevention.

✓   Plaques of atherosclerosis induce hypertension and trigger abnormal blood clotting, leading to heart attacks or strokes. Abnormal vessel spasms can also cause heart attacks and strokes.

✓   Diet-related risk factors for CVD include high LDL and low HDL, hypertension, diabetes, an atherogenic diet , and obesity. The combination of risk factors called metabolic syndrome carries an especially high risk of CVD. Dietary measures to reduce fat, saturated fat, and cholesterol intakes are part of the first line of treatment for high blood cholesterol.

✓   Physical activity can reduce CVD risk. Moderate alcohol intake may also be associated with reduced risk, but its use can be problematic.

✓   Hypertension is silent, progressively worsens atherosclerosis, and makes heart attacks and strokes likely. All adults should know their blood pressure.

✓   Atherosclerosis, obesity, insulin resistance, age, family background, and race contribute to hypertension risks.

✓   For most people, a healthy body weight, regular physical activity, moderation for those who use alcohol, and a diet high in fruits, vegetables, fish and low-fat dairy products and low in fat work together to keep blood pressure normal. For some, salt restriction is also required.

✓   Cancer develops in steps including initiation and promotion, which are thought to be influenced by diet. The body is equipped to handle tiny doses of carcinogens that occur naturally in foods.

✓   Diets high in certain fats and red meats are associated with cancer development. Foods containing fiber, folate, calcium, many other vitamins and minerals, and phytochemicals, along with an ample intake of fluid, are thought to be protective.

Diet and Health

SUMMING UP

The diseases that afflict people around the world are of two main kinds, including infectious

disease and (1) _____ disease. Nutrition can help strengthen the body's defenses

against (2) _____ diseases by supporting a healthy immune system. With respect

to prevention of (3) _____ diseases, choices people make about their nutrition can

help to at least postpone them and sometimes to avoid them altogether.

The body's (4) _____ system guards continuously against disease-

causing agents. Impaired immunity opens the way for diseases, diseases impair (5) _____

assimilation, and nutrition status suffers further. (6) _____ is especially destructive

to various immune system organs and tissues.

People with AIDS and cancer frequently experience malnutrition and

(7) _____ away of the body's tissues. Nutrients cannot cure or reverse the progression

of AIDS, but an adequate diet may help to improve responses to (8) _____

therapy, reduce duration of (9) _____ stays, and promote greater

(10) _____, with an improved quality of life overall.

In contrast to the infectious diseases, the (11) _____ diseases of

adulthood tend to have clusters of suspected contributors known as (12) _____.

Among them are environmental, (13) _____, social, and genetic factors that tend

to occur in clusters and interact with each other. A person who eats a diet high in saturated fat and

calories increases the probabilities of becoming (14) _____ and of contracting

cancer, hypertension, diabetes, atherosclerosis, diverticulosis or other diseases. Many experts

believe that diet accounts for about a (15) _____ of all cases of coronary heart

disease and general trends support the link between diet and (16) _____.

To decide whether certain (17) _____ recommendations are especially

important to you, you should consider your family's (18) _____ history to see

which diseases are common to your forebearers. For example, a person whose close relatives suffered with diabetes and heart disease is advised to avoid becoming (19) _____ and

not to smoke.

In addition to diet, age, cigarette smoking, heart disease or family history of premature

heart disease, diabetes, (20)_____, and physical inactivity predict CVD development.

The big diet-related risk factors for CVD are (21) _____, hypertension, and high

blood (22) _____ and low blood HDL. Generally, cholesterol carried in

(23) _____ correlates directly with risk of heart disease. Dietary measures to

reduce fat, saturated fat, and (24) _____ intakes are part of the first line of

treatment for high blood cholesterol.

Primary among the risk factors that precipitate or aggravate hypertension are

(25)_____, obesity, and (26) _____. Epidemiological studies

have identified several other risk factors that predict hypertension including

(27) _____ and heredity. People with kidney problems or diabetes, those whose

parents have hypertension, African Americans, and persons who are older are especially likely to

be sodium or (28) _____ sensitive.

Some (29) _____ percent of total cancers are influenced by diet. Studies of

populations suggest that low rates of many cancers correlate with intakes of fiber-rich

(30)_____, vegetables and whole grains, particularly (31) _____.

Foods containing fiber, folate, calcium, many other vitamins and minerals, and

(32)_____, along with an ample intake of fluid, are thought to be protective.

CHAPTER GLOSSARY

Matching Exercise:

_____ 1. anticarcinogens

_____ 2. metabolic syndrome

_____ 3. hypertension

_____ 4. carcinogen

_____ 5. plaques

_____ 6. thrombus

_____ 7. metastasis

_____ 8. cruciferous vegetables

_____ 9. atherosclerosis

_____ 10. cancer

_____ 11. calorie effect

_____ 12. heart attack

_____ 13. embolus

_____ 14. aneurysm

_____ 15. initiation

_____ 16. platelets

_____ 17. risk factors

_____ 18. stroke

_____ 19. promoters

a. a disease in which cells multiply out of control and disrupt normal functioning of one or more organs

b. high blood pressure

c. tiny cell-like fragments in the blood, important in blood clot formation

d. a stationary blood clot

e. factors that do not initiate cancer but speed up its development once initiation has taken place

f. a group of vegetables named for their cross-shaped blossoms

g. a thrombus that breaks loose

h. compounds in foods that act in several ways to oppose the formation of cancer

i. the event in which the vessels that feed the heart muscle become closed off by an embolism, thrombus, or other cause with resulting sudden tissue death

j. the sudden shutting off of the blood flow to the brain by a thrombus, embolism, or the bursting of a vessel

k. a cancer-causing substance

l. an event, probably occurring in the cell's genetic material, caused by radiation or by a chemical carcinogen that can give rise to cancer

m. a combination of four risk factors - diabetes, obesity, hypertension, and high blood cholesterol – that greatly increase a person's risk of developing CVD

n. the drop in cancer incidence seen whenever intake of food energy is restricted

o. factors known to be related to (or correlate with) diseases but not proved to be causal

p. mounds of lipid material, mixed with smooth muscle cells and calcium, that develop in the artery walls in atherosclerosis

q. the ballooning out of an artery wall at a point that is weakened by deterioration

r. the most common form of cardiovascular disease, characterized by plaques along the inner walls of the arteries

s. movement of cancer cells from one body part to another, usually by way of the body fluids

EXERCISES

Answer these chapter study questions:

1. Why do malnourished children have repeated lung and digestive tract infections?

2. Why must careful attention be paid to food safety when serving food to people with AIDS?

3. How would you go about deciding whether certain diet recommendations and lifestyle changes are especially important to you?

4. What is the difference between a heart attack and a stroke?

5. Why is it erroneous to think that vitamin supplements can provide all of the benefits of vegetables and fruits as related to cancer prevention?

Complete these short answer questions:

1. These groups of people are especially likely to be caught in the downward spiral of malnutrition and weakened immunity:

    a.
    b
    c.
    d.

2. The major categories of risk factors for degenerative diseases of adulthood include:

    a.
    b
    c.
    d.

3. The big diet-related risk factors for CVD are:

    a.
    b
    c.
    d.

4. The primary risk factors that precipitate or aggravate hypertension are:

    a.
    b
    c.

5. The steps in cancer development are thought to be:

    a.
    b
    c.
    d.
    e.

6. Alcohol intake is associated with cancers of the:

    a.
    b.
    c.

5. The four risk factors that make up the metabolic syndrome include:

    a.
    b.
    c.
    d.

8. Examples of cruciferous vegetables include:

    a.
    b
    c.
    d.
    e.
    f.

9. Ways to minimize risks from carcinogens formed during cooking include:

    a.
    b
    c.
    d.
    e.

10. For most people, these measures work to keep blood pressure normal:

    a.
    b
    c.
    d.

Solve these problems:

1. A serving of a food contains 70 calories and 2 grams of fat. Calculate the percentage of calories from fat in a serving of the food. Would this food be appropriate on a diet in which calories from fat would be 30 percent or less?

2. Jane is a 35 year old who is 65" tall and weighs 130 pounds. She consumes 54 grams of protein, 150 grams of carbohydrate, and 76 grams of fat per day.

    a.   How many calories does Jane consume?

    b.   What is the percent of calories from carbohydrate in Jane's diet and does that amount represent an appropriate diet for disease prevention?

Solve these controversy questions:

1. Which groups of people are most vulnerable to nutrient-drug interactions?

2. How does the overuse of antacids lead to iron deficiency?

3. What type of supplement would you recommend for a woman taking oral contraceptives?

4. How would you define moderation in caffeine intake based on coffee consumption?

5. Why does the vitamin C requirement of smokers exceed that of nonsmokers?

Diet and Health

STUDY AIDS

1. Complete the following table on adult standards for blood pressure, BMI, blood lipids, and risk of CVD.

Blood Pressure

Systolic and diastolic pressure:

130-159/ 85-99 = _____ risk
_____ / _____ = elevated risk

Obesity

Body mass index greater than:_____ = elevated risk

Total Cholesterol

Below _____ mg/dl = low risk
200-239 mg/dl   = _____
_____ mg/dl   = elevated risk

HDL Cholesterol

HDL< _____ mg/dl = elevated risk
≥ 60 mg/dl   = _____ risk

LDL Cholesterol

Below_____ mg/dl = low risk
130-159 mg/dl   = _____
_____ mg/dl   = elevated

Triglycerides (Fasting)

<_____ mg/dl = low risk

2. Use the following table in your textbook as a study aid: Table 11-4 on page 404.

SAMPLE TEST ITEMS

Comprehension Level Items:

1. Nutrition can directly prevent or cure infectious diseases.

    a. true
    b. false

2. Effects of malnutrition on the body's defense systems include:

    a. cells of the immune system are reduced in size
    b. antibody concentration becomes depressed
    c. skin becomes thick with more connective tissue
    d. a and b
    e. b and c

3. A deficiency or a toxicity of even a single nutrient can seriously weaken even a healthy person's immune defense.

    a. true
    b. false

4. Powerful predictors of chronic disease include:

    a. family history
    b. laboratory tests
    c. physical examinations
    d. a and b
    e. a and c

5. Diet is not the only, and perhaps not even the most important, factor in development of CVD.

    a. true
    b. false

6. Which of the following is *not* a major diet-related risk factor for CVD?

    a. diabetes
    b. hypertension
    c. high HDL level
    d. high blood cholesterol

7. To prevent CVD, people in the United States and Canada should:

    a. consume no more than 30% of their calories as fat
    b. consume no more than 20% of their calories as saturated fat
    c. consume no more than 300 milligrams of cholesterol per day
    d. a and b
    e. a and c

8. Which of the following correlates directly with risk of heart disease?

    a. total cholesterol
    b. LDL cholesterol
    c. triglycerides
    d. HDL cholesterol

9. Physical activity and weight loss not only raise HDL concentrations independently of one another, but their effects are additive.

    a. true
    b. false

10. To help lower blood cholesterol you should:

    a. reduce the amount of saturated fat in the diet
    b. shun away from eggs altogether
    c. choose foods high in soluble fiber
    d. a and b
    e. a and c

11. The twin demons that lead to most cardiovascular disease are:

    a. atherosclerosis
    b. hypertension
    c. strokes
    d. a and b
    e. b and c

12. Most people who develop hypertension do so in their:

    a. 20s and 30s
    b. 30s and 40s
    c. 40s and 50s
    d. 50s and 60s

13. The best kind of exercise to reduce hypertension directly is the aerobic kind recommended for cardiovascular endurance.

    a. true
    b. false

14. All of the following are likely to be sodium sensitive individuals *except* for:

    a. those of European or Asian descent
    b. those with kidney problems
    c. those with diabetes
    d. those whose parents have hypertension

15. For about half of people with hypertension, a reduction of blood pressure accompanies a lower salt intake.

    a. true
    b. false

16. For people who are overweight and hypertensive, a loss of _____ pounds may significantly lower blood pressure.

    a. 2
    b. 5
    c. 8
    d. 10

17. Which of the following would you do to consume more phytochemicals in your diet?

    a. eat more fruit
    b. take dietary supplements
    c. use herbs and spices in cooking
    d. a and b
    e. a and c

18. To minimize risks from carcinogens formed during cooking you would:

    a. line the grill with foil
    b. cook foods until they are slightly burned
    c. marinate meats before cooking
    d. a and b
    e. a and c

19. Cruciferous vegetables:

    a. are associated with low cancer rates
    b. include vegetables such as cauliflower, cabbage, and brussels sprouts
    c. contain chemicals that act as promoters of cancer
    d. a and b
    e. b and c

Application Level Items:

20. You are offering help to an AIDS patient. To support his nutrition status you would:

    a. provide three large meals per day
    b. insist that food be consumed rather than supplements
    c. discourage the use of liquid meal replacements
    d. thoroughly cook all foods and practice cleanliness

21. You are concerned that you may be at risk for developing CVD. Which of the following would indicate that you are at risk?

    a. BMI of 30
    b. your father died of a heart attack at age 53
    c. your HDL is 60 mg/dl
    d. a and b
    e. b and c

22. To increase consumption of fiber you would do all of the following *except*:

    a. consume more dried peas and beans
    b. eat more fresh fruit
    c. choose more white breads
    d. eat more whole-grain foods

23. You are a 35 year old male who has just had a physical exam, the results of which are show below. Which of these results indicate that you are at risk for CVD?

    a. blood cholesterol of 180 mg/dl
    b. body mass index of 22
    c. HDL cholesterol of 35 mg/dl
    d. blood pressure of 110/70

24. To decrease your risk of cancer you would:

    a. decrease your intake of fat
    b. increase your intake of smoked foods
    c. eat foods high in fiber
    d. a and b
    e. a and c

25. Henry is interested in reducing his risk for developing hypertension. He should do all of the following *except*:

    a. lose weight if he is overweight
    b. moderate alcohol consumption
    c. decrease his consumption of potassium
    d. moderately restrict salt intake

ANSWERS

SUMMING UP

(1) degenerative; (2) infectious; (3) chronic; (4) immune; (5) food; (6) protein-energy malnutrition; (7) wasting; (8) drug; (9) hospital; (10) independence; (11) degenerative; (12) risk factors; (13) behavioral; (14) obese; (15) third; (16) cancer; (17) diet; (18) medical; (19) obese; (20) obesity; (21) diabetes; (22) LDL; (23) LDL; (24) cholesterol; (25) atherosclerosis; (26) insulin resistance; (27) age; (28) salt; (29) 20-50; (30) fruits; (31) whole wheat; (32) phytochemicals

CHAPTER GLOSSARY

Matching Exercise: (1) h; (2) m; (3) b; (4) k; (5) p; (6) d; (7) s; (8) f; (9) r; (10) a, (11) n; (12) i; (13) g: (14) q; (15) l; (16) c; (17) o; (18) j; (19) e

EXERCISES

Chapter Study Questions:

1. The antibody concentration normally present in secretions of the lungs and digestive tract is depressed in malnutrition which allows infectious agents that would normally be barred from the body to enter. Once they are inside the body, the defense mounted against them is weak.

2. Because a common bacteria in food, such as Salmonella, can cause a deadly infection in people with compromised immunity, such as individuals with AIDS.

3. You should consider your family's medical history to see which diseases are common and also notice which test results are out of line during your physical examination.

4. When an embolus lodges in an artery of the heart and causes sudden death of part of the heart muscle, a heart attack occurs. A stroke occurs when the embolus lodges in an artery of the brain and kills a portion of brain tissue.

5. Although antioxidant nutrients are found in vegetables and fruits, many other nutrients, such as fiber, folate, and calcium are thought to be protective. Vitamin supplements would not supply all of these.

Short Answer Questions:

1. (a) people who restrict their food intake; (b) the very young or old; (c) the hospitalized; (d) the poor

2. (a) environmental; (b) behavioral; (c) social; (d) genetic

3. (a) diabetes; (b) high blood LDL; (c) hypertension; (d) low blood HDL

4.   (a) obesity; (b) atherosclerosis; (c) insulin resistance

5. (a) exposure to a carcinogen; (b) entry of the carcinogen into a cell; (c) initiation; (d) acceleration of other carcinogens called promoters; (e) spreading of cancer cells via blood and lymph

6. (a) mouth; (b) throat; (c) breast

7. (a) diabetes; (b) obesity; (c) hypertension; (d) high blood cholesterol

8. (a) cabbage; (b) cauliflower; (c) broccoli; (d) brussels sprouts; (e) greens; (f) rutabagas

9. (a) wrap food in foil when grilling or line grill with foil; (b) do not burn foods; (c) marinate meats before cooking; (d) limit intake of fried, browned and broiled foods; (e) limit intake of smoked foods

10. (a) healthy body weight; (b) regular physical activity; (c) moderate alcohol intake; (d) diet high in fruits, vegetables, fish and low-fat dairy products and low in fat

Problem-Solving:

1. 26% calories from fat; yes

2. (a) 1500 calories; (b) percentage calories from carbohydrate is 40%; no, because carbohydrates should total more than 55% of calories in a diet for disease prevention

Controversy Questions:

1. Those who take drugs for long times, those who take two or more drugs at the same time, and those who are poorly nourished to begin with or are not eating well.

2. Iron absorbtion is dependent on the stomach's acidity and antacids decrease the acidity and bind with the iron molecules.

3. A standard multivitamin-mineral supplement

4. Two cups of coffee a day

5. Smoking alters the metabolism of vitamin C and smokers break down vitamin C faster and so must take more in to achieve steady body pools comparable to those of nonsmokers

STUDY AIDS

Blood Pressure

Obesity

Systolic and diastolic pressure:

Body mass index greater than: 30 = elevated risk

130-159/ 85-99 = **borderline** risk
$\geq$ **160/ $\geq$100** = elevated risk

Total Cholesterol

HDL Cholesterol

Below **200** mg/dl = low risk
200-239 mg/dl   = **borderline**
$\geq$**240** mg/dl   = elevated risk

HDL< **40** mg/dl = elevated risk
$\geq$ 60 mg/dl   = **low** risk

LDL Cholesterol

Triglycerides (Fasting)

Below **100** mg/dl = low risk
130-159 mg/dl   = **borderline**
160- 189 mg/dl   = elevated

< **150** mg/dl = low risk

SAMPLE TEST ITEMS

1. b (p. 394)	9. a (p. 406)	17. e (p. 417)
2. d (p. 395)	10. e (p. 404-405)	18. e (p. 415)
3. a (p. 396)	11. d (p. 401)	19. d (p. 417)
4. d (p. 398)	12. d (p. 408)	20. d (p. 396)
5. a (p. 401)	13. a (p. 410)	21. d (p. 401-403)
6. c (p. 401)	14. a (p. 409-410)	22. c (p. 415-416)
7. e (p. 404)	15. a (p. 409)	23. c (p. 403)
8. b (p. 403)	16. d (p. 410)	24. e (p. 414-417)
		25. c (p. 409-411)

CHAPTER 12

Life Cycle Nutrition: Mother and Infant

CHAPTER OBJECTIVES

After completing this chapter, you should be able to:

1. Describe how maternal nutrition before and during pregnancy affects both the development of the fetus and growth of the infant after birth.

2. Discuss maternal physiological adjustments that occur during pregnancy and explain how they influence energy and other nutrient requirements.

3. Explain why abstinence from smoking and drugs, avoiding dieting, and moderation in the use of caffeine are recommended during pregnancy.

4. Explain the effects of alcohol on the development of the fetus and describe the condition known as fetal alcohol syndrome.

5. List the benefits of breastfeeding an infant and indicate the changes a lactating woman needs to make in her diet to promote breastfeeding success.

6. Describe the circumstances under which breastfeeding is not recommended and explain what alternatives exist for proper infant nutrition.

7. Plan a timetable for feeding foods to an infant from birth to 12 months of age.

8. Describe what is currently known about relationships between early nutrition and later chronic diseases. (Controversy 12)

KEY CONCEPTS

✓ Adequate nutrition before pregnancy establishes physical readiness and nutrient stores to support fetal growth. Both underweight and overweight women should strive for appropriate body weights before pregnancy. Newborns who weigh less that 5 1/2 pounds face greater health risks than normal-weight babies. The healthy development of the placenta depends on adequate nutrition before pregnancy.

✓ Placental development, implantation, and early critical periods depend on maternal nutrition before and during pregnancy.

✓ Pregnancy brings physiological adjustments that demand increased intakes of energy and nutrients. A daily iron supplement is recommended for all pregnant women during the second and third trimesters. Food assistance programs such as WIC can benefit pregnant women of limited financial means.

✓ Weight gain is essential for a healthy pregnancy. A woman's prepregnancy BMI, her own nutrient needs, and the number of fetuses she is carrying help to determine an appropriate weight gain.

✓ Physically fit women can continue to be physically active throughout pregnancy. Pregnant women should be cautious in their choice of activities.

✓ Of all the population groups, pregnant teenage girls have the highest nutrient needs and an increased likelihood of having problem pregnancies.

✓ Food cravings usually do not reflect physiological needs, and some may interfere with nutrition. Nausea arises from normal hormonal changes of pregnancy.

✓ Abstaining from smoking and other drugs, limiting intake of foods known to contain unsafe levels of contaminants such as mercury, avoiding large doses of nutrients, refraining from dieting, and limiting caffeine use are recommended during pregnancy.

✓ Alcohol limits oxygen delivery to the fetus, slows cell division, and reduces the number of cells organs produce. Alcoholic beverages must bear warnings to pregnant women.

✓ The birth defects of fetal alcohol syndrome arise from severe damage to the fetus caused by alcohol. Lesser conditions, ARND and ARBD, may be harder to diagnose, but also rob the child of a normal life.

✓ Abstinence from alcohol is critical to prevent irreversible damage to the fetus.

✓ Common medical problems associated with pregnancy are gestational diabetes and preeclampsia. These should be managed to minimize associated risks.

✓ The lactating woman needs extra fluid and enough energy and nutrients to make sufficient milk each day. Malnutrition most often diminishes the quantity of the milk produced without altering quality. Lactation facilitates loss of the extra fat gained during pregnancy.

✓ Breastfeeding is inadvisable if the mother's milk is contaminated with alcohol, drugs or environmental pollutants. Most ordinary infections such as colds have no effect on breastfeeding. The decision to breastfeed or not in the case of an HIV-infected woman depends on availability of formula and clean water.

✓ Infants' rapid growth and development depend heavily on adequate nutrient supplies. Adequate water is also crucial.

✓ Breast milk is the ideal food for infants, with the needed nutrients in the right proportions and also protective factors. It is especially valuable for premature infants.

✓ Infant formulas are designed to resemble breast milk and must meet an AAP standard for nutrient composition. Special formulas are available for premature babies, allergic babies, and others. Formula should be replaced with milk only after the baby's first birthday.

✓ Solid food additions to a baby's diet should begin at about six months and should be governed by the baby's nutrient needs and readiness to eat. By one year, the baby should be receiving foods from all food groups.

✓ The early feeding of the infant lays the foundation for lifelong eating habits. It is desirable to foster preferences that will support normal development throughout life.

SUMMING UP

Before she becomes pregnant, a woman must establish eating habits that will optimally

(1) _____ both the growing fetus and herself and strive for an appropriate body

(2) _____. An underweight woman who fails to gain adequately during pregnancy

is most likely to bear a baby with a dangerously low (3) _____. Infant birthweight

is the most potent single indicator of an infant's future (4) _____ status. Prepregnancy

nutrition determines whether the woman will be able to grow a healthy

(5) _____, which is the only source of (6) _____ available to the fetus.

During the two weeks following fertilization, minimal growth takes place but it is a

(7) _____ period developmentally. At eight weeks, the fetus has a complete

central nervous system, a beating (8) _____, and a fully formed (9) _____

system. The gestation period, which lasts approximately (10) _____ weeks, ends

with the (11) _____ of the infant.

Pregnancy requires only (12) _____ extra calories per day above the

allowance for nonpregnant women. In addition, about (13) _____ grams of

protein are required. Pregnant women need generous amounts of (14) _____ -rich

foods to spare their protein and to provide energy. Vitamins needed in large amounts during

pregnancy include (15) _____ and vitamin B_{12}. Calcium, (16) _____,

and magnesium are the minerals in greatest demand during pregnancy. Although the body

conserves (17) _____ even more than usual during pregnancy, an iron supplement

is recommended during the second and third trimesters. The ideal pattern of weight gain is

thought to be 2 to 4 pounds during the first (18) _____ months and a

(19) _____ per week thereafter.

The energy cost of producing milk is about (20) _____ calories a day.

The nursing mother should drink at least (21) _____ quarts of liquids each day to

prevent dehydration. Breastfeeding may be inadvisable if milk is contaminated with

(22) _____ , drugs, or environmental pollutants.

The most important nutrient for infants is (23) _____ and

(24) _____ milk is considered the most desirable source of nutrients for the young

infant. With respect to nutrient needs during infancy, the nutrient needed most is

(25) _____, then vitamin (26) _____ .

Solid food additions to a baby's diet should begin at about (27) _____

months and should be governed by the baby's nutrient needs and (28) _____ to

eat. The early feeding of an infant should foster preferences that will support normal

(29)_____ and health throughout life and help avert common

(30) _____ diseases.

CHAPTER GLOSSARY

Matching Exercise 1:

_____ 1. critical period	a. the stage of human gestation from the third to eighth week after conception
_____ 2. gestation	b. a system of scoring an infant's physical condition right after birth
_____ 3. amniotic sac	c. the period of about 40 weeks (three trimesters) from conception to birth; the term of a pregnancy
_____ 4. fetus	d. the stage of human gestation from eight weeks after conception until birth of an infant
_____ 5. ovum	e. a birthweight of less than 5 1/2 pounds (2,500 grams); used as a predictor of probable health problems in the newborn and as a probable indicator of poor nutrition status of the mother before and/or during pregnancy
_____ 6. embryo	
_____ 7. zygote	f. the womb, the muscular organ within which the infant develops before birth
_____ 8. uterus	g. a finite period during development in which certain events may occur that will have irreversible effects on later developmental stages
_____ 9. placenta	
_____ 10. Apgar score	h. the stage of development, during the first two weeks after conception, in which the fertilized egg embeds itself in the wall of the uterus and begins to develop
_____ 11. implantation	i. the term that describes the product of the union of ovum and sperm during the first two weeks after fertilization
_____ 12. low birthweight	
_____ 13. Special Supplemental Food Program for Women, Infants, and Children (WIC)	j. the organ that develops inside the uterus in early pregnancy in which maternal and fetal blood circulate in close proximity and exchange materials
	k. the egg, produced by the mother, that unites with a sperm from the father to produce a new individual
	l. the "bag of waters" in the uterus in which the fetus floats
_____ 14. environmental tobacco smoke	m. a condition caused by prenatal alcohol exposure; diagnosed when there is a history of substantial regular maternal alcohol intake or heavy episodic drinking, combined with birth defects known to be associated with alcohol exposure
_____ 15. alcohol-related birth defects (ARBD)	
	n. the combination of exhaled smoke (mainstream smoke) and smoke from lighted cigarettes, pipes, or cigars (sidestream smoke) that enters the air and may be inhaled by other people.
	o. a USDA program to provide nutrition support to low-income women who are pregnant or have infants or preschool children

Matching Exercise 2:

_____ 1. preeclampsia

_____ 2. neural tube defects

_____ 3. colostrum

_____ 4. spina bifida

_____ 5. edema

_____ 6. alpha-lactalbumin

_____ 7. lactoferrin

_____ 8. anencephaly

_____ 9. gestational diabetes

_____ 10. fetal alcohol syndrome

_____ 11. lactation

_____ 12. milk anemia

_____ 13. cesarean section

_____ 14. alcohol-related neurodevelopmental disorder (ARND)

a. the chief protein in human breast milk

b. abnormal glucose tolerance appearing during pregnancy, with subsequent return to normal after the end of pregnancy

c. production and secretion of breast milk for the purpose of nourishing an infant

d. a group of nervous system abnormalities caused by interruption of the normal early development of the neural tube

e. accumulation of fluid in the tissues

f. a severe neural tube defect in which the brain fails to form

g. a milklike secretion from the breast during the first day or so after delivery before milk appears

h. a potentially dangerous condition during pregnancy characterized by edema, hypertension, and protein in the urine

i. the cluster of symptoms seen in an infant or child whose mother consumed excessive alcohol during her pregnancy

j. iron-deficiency anemia caused by drinking so much milk that iron-rich foods are displaced from the diet

k. a type of neural tube defect in which infants are born with gaps in the bones of the spine, leaving the spinal cord protected only by a sheath of skin in those spots, or with no protection at all

l. a factor in breast milk that binds iron and keeps it from supporting the growth of the infant's intestinal bacteria

m. a condition caused by prenatal alcohol exposure; diagnosed when there is a confirmed history of substantial regular maternal alcohol intake or heavy episodic drinking, combined with behavioral, cognitive, or central nervous system abnormalities in the child that are known to be associated with alcohol exposure

n. surgical childbirth, in which the infant is taken through an incision in the woman's abdomen

EXERCISES

Answer these chapter study questions:

1. Why is an appropriate prepregnancy weight important and how does it relate to pregnancy outcome?

2. Do all women need to add protein-rich foods to their diets in order to obtain the additional daily protein recommended during pregnancy? Why or why not?

3. How does a woman's body conserve iron during pregnancy? Does this mean that an iron supplement should not be taken?

4. What effect does nutritional deprivation of the mother have on breastfeeding?

5. Discuss ways to prevent infant obesity and to encourage eating habits that will support continued normal weight as the child grows.

Complete these short answer questions:

1. Factors associated with low-birthweight infants include:

   a.
   b.
   c.
   d.
   e.

2. The effects of malnutrition during critical periods of pregnancy are seen in:

   a.
   b.
   c.

3. The pregnant woman's need for folate increases from 400 to 600 micrograms/day due to:

   a.
   b.

4. These minerals, involved in building the skeleton, are in great demand during pregnancy:

   a.
   b.
   c.

5. Nutrient supplements needed for pregnant women at nutritional risk include:

   a.   e.
   b.   f.
   c.   g.
   d.   h.

6. Components of weight gained by the pregnant woman include these lean tissues:

    a.
    b.
    c.
    d.
    e.

7. The nausea of morning sickness can be alleviated by starting the day with:

    a.
    b.

8. Supplemental water should be provided to an infant on infant formula or breast milk under the following conditions:

    a.
    b.
    c.
    d.

9. The addition of foods to a baby's diet should be governed by these three conditions:

    a.
    b.
    c.

10. Normal dental development in a baby should be promoted by:

    a.
    b.
    c.
    d.

Solve these problems:

1. Calculate the caloric needs and grams of carbohydrate and protein which should be provided in a diet for a 30 year old pregnant woman who weighs 130 pounds and is at her appropriate weight for height. Her nonpregnant caloric needs are 2000 calories per day.

For questions 2-6, match the nutrients needed in extra amounts during pregnancy, listed on the right, with some of their best food sources, listed on the left.

_____2. dried fruits   a. folate

_____3. dark, green leafy vegetables b. calcium

_____4. eggs   c. iron

_____5. milk   d. zinc

_____6. shellfish   e. vitamin B_{12}

For questions 7-12, identify the correct sequence for introducing the following foods into an infant's diet, by placing an "*a*" by the first food which should be introduced, a "*b*" by the second food to be introduced, etc.

_____ 7. pureed vegetables

_____ 8. pieces of soft, cooked vegetables from the table

_____ 9. yogurt

_____10. iron-fortified rice cereal

_____11. mashed fruits

_____12. finely-chopped meat

Solve these controversy questions:

1. What is meant by the "*fetal origins*" hypothesis?

2. What are common conditions and diseases associated with the diagnosis of type 2 diabetes in children?

3. What are characteristics of physically active children versus sedentary children?

4. What are appropriate dietary guidelines for children found to have high blood lipids?

5. Describe the characteristics of children most likely to develop type 2 diabetes.

STUDY AIDS

Complete the following table by filling in the blanks.

First Foods for the Infant

Age (months)	*Addition*
0-4	Breast milk or (a) _____
4-6	Iron fortified (b) _____ mixed with breast milk, formula, or water
6-8	Begin (c) _____ and other cereals and mashed (d) _____ and fruits
8-10	Begin yogurt, finely cut (e) _____, fish, casseroles, cheese, (f) _____, and legumes

Use the following tables in your textbook as study aids: Table 12-2 on page 441; Table 12-5 on page 444; Table 12-8 on page 458.

SAMPLE TEST ITEMS

Comprehension Level Items:

1. Which of the following is the major factor in low birthweight?

    a. heredity
    b. smoking
    c. drug use
    d. poor nutrition

2. The muscular organ within which the infant develops before birth is called:

    a. placenta
    b. uterus
    c. ovum
    d. zygote

3. The stage of human gestation from the third to eighth week after conception is called a(an):

    a. ovum
    b. zygote
    c. embryo
    d. fetus

4. The recommended protein intake during pregnancy is _____ grams per day.

    a. 45
    b. 50
    c. 60
    d. 100

5. Folic acid, the synthetic form of folate, is better absorbed than the naturally occurring folate in foods.

    a. true
    b. false

6. A daily iron supplement containing _____ milligrams is recommended during the second and third trimesters of pregnancy.

    a. 10
    b. 20
    c. 30
    d. 40

7. A sudden large weight gain during pregnancy is a signal that may indicate:

   a. that the woman is consuming too many calories
   b. that the baby will be too large
   c. the onset of preeclampsia
   d. a and b
   e. b and c

8. Which of the following practices should be avoided during pregnancy?

   a. exercise
   b. dieting
   c. consumption of caffeine
   d. a and b
   e. b and c

9. A strategy which has been found effective in alleviating the nausea of morning sickness is to start the day with:

   a. a few sips of lemonade
   b. a food high in fat
   c. a salty snack food
   d. a and b
   e. a and c

10. Breast milk volume depends on:

    a. the size of the mother's breasts
    b. how much fluid the mother consumes
    c. how much milk the baby demands
    d. a and b
    e. b and c

11. Characteristics of breast milk include all of the following *except*:

    a. it has a 2-to-1 calcium-to-phosphorus ratio
    b. it is high in sodium
    c. its iron is highly absorbable
    d. its zinc is absorbed better than from cow's milk

12. A baby less than one year of age who has been on breast milk should be weaned onto:

    a. whole milk
    b. skim milk
    c. low-fat milk
    d. infant formula

13. Which of the following ranks highest on the list of nutrients most needing attention in infant nutrition?

    a. vitamin C
    b. vitamin D
    c. iron
    d. vitamin A

14. Food aversions and cravings that arise during pregnancy are usually due to:

    a. changes in taste
    b. physiological needs
    c. changes in smell sensitivities
    d. a and b
    e. a and c

15. Birth defects have been observed in the children of some women who drank
    _____ounces of alcohol daily during pregnancy.

    a. 2
    b. 3
    c. 4
    d. 5

16. Producing 25 ounces of milk a day costs a woman almost _____calories per day.

    a. 300
    b. 525
    c. 650
    d. 1000

17. The birthweight of an infant triples by the age of:

    a. 4 months
    b. 6 months
    c. 9 months
    d. 1 year

18. Supplements of these nutrients may be necessary for a breastfed infant:

    a. vitamin C, calcium, and iron
    b. vitamin D, fluoride, and iron
    c. magnesium, zinc, and calcium
    d. vitamin C, zinc, and fluoride

19. Water should be offered to infants regularly once they are eating solid foods.

    a. true
    b. false

Application Level Items:

20. Lola experienced malnutrition late in her pregnancy. Which of the following organs of the infant will most likely be affected?

    a. heart
    b. lungs
    c. brain
    d. a and c
    e. b and c

21. Cindy is a 25 year old pregnant female who recently experienced a sudden weight gain. In addition, she has blurred vision, is dizzy, and has frequent headaches. Cindy is most likely experiencing symptoms of:

    a. malnutrition
    b. gestational diabetes
    c. preeclampsia
    d. a normal pregnancy

22. A nonpregnant woman requires 2200 calories to maintain her desirable body weight. How many calories would she need if she became pregnant?

    a. 2100
    b. 2300
    c. 2500
    d. 2750

23. How many grams of carbohydrate are needed by a pregnant woman consuming 2500 calories per day?

    a. 138
    b. 182
    c. 275
    d. 313

24. Jane weighs 160 pounds and is considered to be overweight. Approximately how much should Jane weigh at the end of her pregnancy?

    a. 160
    b. 173
    c. 180
    d. 190

25. Which of the following indicates an infant who is ready for solid foods?

    a. Jeff, who is 4 months old
    b. Claudia, who can sit with support and control head movements
    c. Ben, who swallows using the back of his tongue
    d. Sarah, who turns her head toward any object that brushes her cheek

ANSWERS

SUMMING UP

(1) nourish; (2) weight; (3) birthweight; (4) health; (5) placenta; (6) sustenance; (7) critical;
(8) heart; (9) digestive; (10) 40; (11) birth; (12) 300; (13) 60; (14) carbohydrate; (15) folate;
(16) phosphorus; (17) iron; (18) three; (19) pound; (20) 650; (21) two; (22) alcohol; (23) water;
(24) breast; (25) iron; (26) C; (27) six; (28) readiness; (29) development; (30) lifestyle

CHAPTER GLOSSARY

Matching Exercise 1: *(1)* g; (2) c; (3) l; (4) d; (5) k; (6) a; (7) i; (8) f; (9) j; (10) b; (11) h;
(12) e; (13) o; (14) n; (15) m
Matching Exercise 2: *(1)* h; (2) d; (3) g; (4) k; (5) e; (6) a; (7) l; (8) f; (9) b; (10) i; (11) c;
(12) j; (13) n; (14) m

EXERCISES

Chapter Study Questions:

1. A strong correlation exists between prepregnancy weight, weight gain during pregnancy, and infant birthweight. Infant birthweight is the most potent single indication of the infant's future health status. Low birthweight babies have a greater chance of dying early in life and of having illnesses.

2. No; many women in the United States exceed the recommended protein intake for pregnancy even when they are not pregnant and excessive protein intake may have adverse effects.

3. Menstruation ceases and the absorption of iron increases up to threefold. However, because iron stores dwindle, the maternal blood volume increases, and few women enter pregnancy with adequate stores to meet pregnancy demands, a supplement is recommended during the second and third trimesters.

4. In general, the effect of nutritional deprivation is to reduce the quantity, not the quality, of milk. However, the levels of fat-soluble vitamins in human milk can be affected by excessive or deficient intakes of the mother.

5. A variety of nutritious foods should be introduced in an inviting way; the baby should not be forced to finish a bottle or jar of baby food; concentrated sweets and empty-calorie foods should be limited; babies should not be taught to seek food as a reward and they should not be comforted or punished with food.

Short Answer Questions:

1. (a) poor nutrition; (b) heredity; (c) disease conditions; (d) smoking; (e) drug use

2. (a) neural tube defects of the nervous system of the embryo; (b) poor dental health of children whose mothers were malnourished during pregnancy; (c) adult's vulnerability to infections and possibly higher risks of diabetes, hypertension, stroke and heart disease

3. (a) the great increase in the number of the mother's red blood cells; (b) new cells being laid down at a tremendous pace as the fetus grows and develops

4. (a) calcium; (b) phosphorus; (c) magnesium

5. (a) folate; (b) vitamin B_6; (c) vitamin C; (d) vitamin D; (e) calcium; (f) copper; (g) iron; (h) zinc

6. (a) placenta; (b) uterus; (c) blood; (d) milk-producing glands; (e) fetus itself

7. (a) a few sips of a carbonated drink; (b) a few nibbles of soda crackers or other salty snack foods

8. (a) hot weather; (b) diarrhea; (c) vomiting; (d) sweating

9. (a) the baby's nutrient needs; (b) the baby's physical readiness to handle different forms of foods; (c) need to detect and control allergic reactions

10. (a) supplying nutritious foods; (b) avoiding sweets; (c) discouraging the association of food with reward or comfort; (d) discouraging the use of a bottle as a pacifier

Problem-Solving:

1. (a) caloric needs: 2000 calories + 300 calories = 2300 calories; (b) recommended carbohydrate intake = 50% of calories; 2300 x 50% = 1150 calories = 288 grams carbohydrate; (c) recommended protein intake = 60 grams
2. c
3. a
4. e
5. b
6. d
7. b
8. e
9. d
10. a
11. c
12. f

Controversy Questions:

1. The hypothesis proposes that fetal nutrition may change development in ways that last a lifetime

2. Type 2 diabetes in children is associated with obesity, hypertension, elevated blood lipids, and cardiovascular disease

3. Physically active children have higher HDL, lower LDL, and lower blood pressure than sedentary children

4. A diet that meets recommendations of the Dietary Guidelines for reducing fat, saturated fat, and cholesterol and increasing fiber while following the Food Guide Pyramid for adequacy

5. They are overweight, female, have a family history of type 2 diabetes, of non-European descent, born to mothers who had diabetes while pregnant with them, and have insulin resistance

STUDY AIDS

1. (a) infant formula; (b) cereal; (c) breads; (d) vegetables; (e) meats; (f) eggs

SAMPLE TEST ITEMS

1. d (p. 436)	9. c (p. 446)	17. d (p. 455)
2. b (p. 437)	10. c (p. 452)	18. b (p. 458)
3. c (p. 438)	11. b (p. 457-458)	19. a (p. 461)
4. c (p. 439)	12. d (p. 459)	20. b (p. 439)
5. a (p. 442)	13. c (p. 461)	21. c (p. 451-452)
6. c (p. 443)	14. e (p. 446)	22. c (p. 439)
7. c (p. 444)	15. a (p. 449)	23. d (p. 440)
8. b (p. 446-448)	16. c (p. 452)	24. c (p. 444)
		25. b (p. 461-463)

CHAPTER 13

Child, Teen, and Older Adult

CHAPTER OBJECTIVES

After completing this chapter, you should be able to:

1. Describe the nutrient needs of young children and appropriate feeding practices including such issues as choking, portion sizes, and snacking.

2. Discuss nutrition-related concerns of children including the link between diet and behavior, the problem of lead, and the impact of television on nutrition.

3. Distinguish between food allergies, intolerances, and aversions.

4. Discuss the special nutrient needs and concerns of teenagers including the effect of diet on PMS and acne.

5. Discuss special nutritional needs of older adults and the suspected connections between diet and disease.

6. Discuss the relationship between food, mind, and memory. (Controversy 13)

KEY CONCEPTS

✓ Children's nutrient needs reflect their stage of growth. For a healthy child, use the Food Guide Pyramid for Young Children and the Dietary Guidelines for Americans as guides. Positive parental guidance can help establish food patterns that provide adequate nourishment for growth without obesity.

✓ Healthy eating habits and positive relationships with food are learned in childhood. Parents teach children best by example. Choking hazards can often be avoided.

✓ The detrimental effects of nutrient deficiencies in children in developed nations can be subtle. Iron deficiency is the most widespread nutrition problem of children and causes abnormalities in both physical health and behavior. Iron toxicity is a major form of poisoning in children.

✓ Lead poisoning has declined dramatically over the past two decades, but it can inflict severe, irreparable damage on growing children. Higher awareness of the remaining sources of lead poisoning can help to reduce the present rate of occurrence.

✓ Food allergies cause illness, but diagnosis is difficult. Tests are imperative to determine whether allergy exists. Food aversions can be related to food allergies or to adverse reactions to food.

✓ Hyperactivity, properly named attention-deficit/hyperactivity disorder (ADHD), is not caused by food or poor nutrition; temporary "*hyper*" behavior may reflect excess caffeine consumption or inconsistent care. A wise parent will limit children's caffeine intakes and meet their needs for structure to prevent tension and fatigue.

✓ The nation's children are growing fatter and face growing risks of disease. Childhood obesity demands careful family-centered management. Television viewing can contribute to obesity through lack of exercise and promoting overconsumption of calorie-dense snacks. Such snacks may also contribute to dental caries.

✓ Breakfast is critical to school performance. Not all children start the day with an adequate breakfast, but school breakfast programs help to fill the need.

✓ School lunches are designed to provide at least a third of the daily nutrients needed by growing children and to stay within limits set by the Dietary Guidelines for Americans. Sodas and snack vending machines, fast-food, snack bars, and school stores tempt school children with foods high in fats and sugars. Fruit juice is a healthy food, but may cause dental problems if used to excess.

✓ Growth patterns and nutrient and energy needs of teens vary widely with gender, body size, and activity level.

✓ With planning, the gatekeeper can encourage teens to meet nutrient requirements by providing nutritious snacks.

✓ Although no foods have been proven to aggravate acne, stress can worsen it. Supplements are useless against acne, but sunlight, proven medications and relief from stress can help.

✓ Life expectancy for U.S. adults increased in the twentieth century. No specific diet or supplement is proved to prolong human life.

✓ Energy needs decrease with age, but exercise burns off excess fuel, maintains lean tissue, and brings health benefits.

✓ Generous carbohydrate intakes are recommended for older adults. Including fiber in the diet is important to avoid constipation.

✓ A diet high in fruits and vegetables and low in fats of meats and dairy products may improve some symptoms of arthritis. Omega-3 fatty acids may also have a positive effect.

✓ Protein needs remain about the same through adult life, but choosing low-fat fiber-rich protein foods may help control other health problems.

✓ Vitamin A absorption increases with aging. Older people suffer more from deficiencies of vitamin D and vitamin B_{12} than young people do. Cataracts and macular degeneration often occur among those with low fruit and vegetable intakes.

✓ Aging alters vitamin and mineral needs. Some needs rise while others decline.

✓ Lifestyle factors can make a difference in aging. In rats, food energy deprivation may lengthen the lives of individuals who survive the treatment. Claims for life extension through antioxidants or other supplements are common hoaxes.

✓ Alzheimer's disease causes some degree of brain deterioration in as many as one-fifth of people past age 65. Current treatment helps only marginally; dietary aluminum is probably unrelated. Nutrition care gains importance as the disease progresses.

✓ Food choices of the elderly are affected by aging, altered health status, and changed life circumstances. Assistance programs can help by providing nutritious meals, providing social interactions, and easing financial problems.

SUMMING UP

Nutrient needs change throughout life and vary depending on the rate of growth,

(1) _____, activities, and many other factors. An infant's appetite decreases near the

(2) _____ birthday, in line with the great reduction in growth rate. A one year old child

needs about (3) _____ calories a day; a three year old needs only (4) _____

calories more. Before their adolescent growth spurt, children accumulate stores of

(5) _____ that they will need in the years ahead.

     "*Hyper*" behavior in children may reflect excess (6) _____ consumption

or inconsistent care. Excess caffeine may be consumed by children in the form of tempting

(7) _____ and chocolate. Research has found that obesity in children may be related to (8) _____ viewing, which affects children's nutritional health adversely in several ways.

   With the onset of (9) _____, needs for all nutrients become greater than at any other time of life except during pregnancy and lactation. In females, (10) _____ becomes a larger percentage of the total body weight. On the average, about a fourth of a teenager's total daily energy intake comes from (11) _____. One of the many changes girls face as they become women is the onset of (12) _____. The hormones that regulate the menstrual cycle also alter metabolic rate, glucose tolerance, (13) _____, food intake, mood, and (14) _____.

   Teenagers often fail to obtain enough vitamin (15) _____ and iron. Another problem nutrient for teenagers is (16) _____, which may fall short unless they snack on dairy products. Although no foods have been proven to aggravate acne, (17) _____ can worsen it.

   In the U.S., the life expectancy at birth is (18) _____ years for white women and 75 years for white men. Nutrient needs become more individual with age, depending on genetics and medical history, but (19) _____ needs often decrease with advancing age. Generous (20) _____ intakes are recommended for older adults and a diet high in fruits and vegetables and low in (21) _____ of meats and dairy products may improve some symptoms of arthritis.

   (22) _____is a major risk for older adults, who may not notice or pay attention to their thirst. With age, (23) _____ takes on extra importance for its role against constipation. Among the vitamins, vitamin (24) _____stands alone in that absorption appears to increase with aging. Older adults also face a greater risk of vitamin (25) _____ deficiency than younger people do. Cataracts are more likely to occur in people with low fruit and green (26) _____ intakes. Iron deficiency is less common in older adults than in

younger people, but (27) _____ deficiencies are common in older people and may lead

to decreased appetite and a diminished sense of (28) _____.

CHAPTER GLOSSARY

Matching Exercise:

_____ 1. premenstrual syndrome

_____ 2. puberty

_____ 3. anaphylactic shock

_____ 4. food aversion

_____ 5. allergy

_____ 6. longevity

_____ 7. senile dementia

_____ 8. life span

_____ 9. hyperactivity

_____ 10. life expectancy

_____ 11. acne

_____ 12. histamine

_____ 13. antigen

_____ 14. cataracts

_____ 15. food intolerance

_____ 16. antibodies

_____ 17. arthritis

_____ 18. learning disability

_____ 19. epiphyseal plate

a. a syndrome characterized by inattention, impulsiveness, and excess motor activity

b. a life-threatening whole-body allergic reaction to an offending substance

c. an adverse effect of a food or food additive not involving the immune response

d. an immune reaction to a foreign substance, such as a component of food

e. a substance foreign to the body that elicits the formation of antibodies or an inflammation reaction from immune system cells

f. a cluster of symptoms that some women experience prior to and during menstruation

g. the loss of brain function beyond the normal loss of physical adeptness and memory that occurs with aging

h. a chronic inflammation of the skin's follicles and oil-producing glands, which leads to an accumulation of oils inside the ducts that surround hairs

i. large protein molecules that are produced in response to the presence of antigens and then help to inactivate the antigens

j. the period in life when a person develops sexual maturity and the ability to reproduce

k. a substance produced by cells of the immune system as part of a local immune reaction to an antigen

l. an intense dislike of a food, possibly biological in nature, resulting from an illness or other negative experience associated with that food

m. the average number of years lived by people in a given society

n. thickening of the lens of the eye that can lead to blindness

o. long duration of life

p. a usually painful inflammation of the joints caused by many conditions, including infections, metabolic disturbances, or injury

q. the maximum number of years of life attainable by a member of a species

r. a thick cartilage-like layer that forms new cells that are eventually calcified, lengthening the bone

s. any of a group of conditions resulting in an altered ability to learn basic cognitive skills such as reading, writing, and mathematics

EXERCISES

Answer these chapter study questions:

1. Identify four ways in which television affects children's nutritional health adversely.

2. Compare the characteristics of children who eat no breakfast with those of their well-fed peers.

3. What recommendations would you make to an individual who experiences PMS?

4. Why should fats be limited in the diets of older adults?

5. Why do energy needs decrease with age?

Complete these short answer questions:

1. School lunches must include specified servings of:

    a.
    b.
    c.
    d.
    e.

2. Allergies may have these one or two components:

    a.
    b.

3. The life threatening food allergy reaction of anaphylactic shock is most often caused by these foods:

    a.   e.
    b.   f.
    c.   g.
    d.   h.

4. Normal, everyday causes of *"hyper"* behavior in children include:

    a.
    b.
    c.
    d.
    e.
    f.
    g.

5. Hormones that regulate the menstrual cycle also alter:

   a.
   b.
   c.
   d.
   e.
   f.

6. Deficiencies of these minerals enhance lead absorption:

   a.
   b.
   c.
   d.
   e.

7. Minerals frequently lacking in older people's diets include:

   a.
   b.
   c.

8. Older people face a greater risk of vitamin D deficiency than younger people do because:

   a.
   b.
   c.

9. Six factors that affect physiological age include:

   a.
   b.
   c.
   d.
   e.
   f.

10. This cluster of symptoms justifies a diagnosis of Alzheimer's Disease:

   a.
   b.
   c.

Solve these problems:

1. Below is a sample day's menu for a 4-6 year old child. Compare the menu with the Food
    Guide Pyramid for Young Children and identify foods and potential nutrients which would be
    missing from the child's diet.

    ### Menu

    Breakfast: Cheese toast with 1 slice of whole-wheat bread and 1 ounce of cheddar cheese; 3/4
    cup orange juice; 1/2 cup whole milk

    Lunch: Peanut butter and jelly sandwich with 4 tbsp. peanut butter and 2 tbsp. jelly on 2
    slices of whole-wheat bread; 1 apple; 1 cup whole milk

    Dinner: 2 ounces of steak; 1/2 cup mashed potato with 1 tbsp. butter; 1 dinner roll; 1 cup
    strawberry yogurt

    Snack: 3 chocolate chip cookies

2. Identify whether the following foods have high or low caries potential by placing an x in the
    appropriate space.

	Low Caries Potential	High Caries Potential
a. plain yogurt	_____	_____
b. sugared cereals	_____	_____
c. bagels	_____	_____
d. dried fruit	_____	_____
e. popcorn	_____	_____
f. glazed carrots	_____	_____
g. sugarless gum	_____	_____
h. legumes	_____	_____
i. fresh fruit	_____	_____
j. chocolate milk	_____	_____

3. For each nutrient listed below, indicate whether nutritional needs for older adults are higher,
    lower, or the same as that for younger adults.

	Higher	Lower	Same
a. energy	_____	_____	_____
b. fiber	_____	_____	_____
c. vitamin A	_____	_____	_____
d. vitamin D	_____	_____	_____
e. protein	_____	_____	_____

Solve these controversy questions:

1. What happens when the blood delivers too little oxygen or glucose to the brain?

2. Which dietary components raise or lower the brain's concentration of serotonin?

3. How does dieting disrupt mental functioning?

4. Which of the brain's principal neurotransmitters has been associated with depression?

5. What dietary suggestion would you offer to a classmate who tends to nod off during exams?

STUDY AIDS

Use the following figure and table in your textbook as study aids: Figure 13-1 on page 475; Table 13-8 on page 496 .

SAMPLE TEST ITEMS

Comprehension Level Items:

1. The most common nutrient deficiency among children and adolescents in the United States is:

    a.   calcium deficiency
    b.   iron deficiency
    c.   vitamin D deficiency
    d.   vitamin A deficiency

2. Television's influence on nutrition is evident in:

    a.   childhood obesity
    b.   dental health of children
    c.   childhood eating disorders
    d.   a and b
    e.   b and c

3. Which of the following foods most often cause allergic reactions?

    a.   cheese
    b.   poultry
    c.   peanuts
    d.   rye

4. Which of the following is true of children who eat no breakfast compared to those who do?

    a.   they perform poorly in tasks of concentration
    b.   their attention spans are longer
    c.   they achieve higher test scores than their well-fed peers
    d.   they have higher rates of obesity than their well-fed peers

5. Needs for all nutrients are greater during _____ than at any other time of life except during pregnancy and lactation.

    a.   infancy
    b.   childhood
    c.   adolescence
    d.   adulthood

6. On the average, approximately one-fourth of teenagers' total daily energy intake comes from:

   a. snacks
   b. the school lunch program
   c. meals
   d. fast food meals

7. To get children to accept vegetables you would:

   a. serve vegetables which are easy to eat
   b. serve vegetables that are highly flavored
   c. serve brightly colored vegetables
   d. a and b
   e. a and c

8. Prevention of lead toxicity in children rests primarily on:

   a. reduced exposure
   b. adequate intake of calcium
   c. increased awareness of mothers
   d. adequate intake of iron

9. Which of the following foods have been shown not to worsen acne?

   a. chocolate
   b. fatty acids
   c. sugar
   d. a and b
   e. a and c

10. Which of the following would you recommend to a woman who experiences PMS?

    a. a diuretic
    b. vitamin E supplement
    c. a caffeine-free lifestyle
    d. a fiber restricted diet

11. Which of the following protein sources would you recommend to an older adult with constipation?

    a. beef
    b. eggs
    c. legumes
    d. milk

12. In the United States, the life expectancy for black men is:

    a. 68 years
    b. 79 years
    c. 80 years
    d. 115 years

13. A diet low in _____ may improve some symptoms of arthritis.

    a. protein
    b. sodium
    c. sugar
    d. fat

14. Energy needs often decrease with advancing age.

    a. true
    b. false

15. As a person grows older:

    a. dehydration becomes a major risk
    b. fiber takes on extra importance
    c. protein needs increase
    d. a and b
    e. b and c

16. Which of the following statements is true concerning the dietary habits of older adults?

    a. they have cut down on saturated fats
    b. they are eating fewer vegetables
    c. they are consuming more milk
    d. they are eating fewer whole-grain breads

17. There is an apparent increase in the absorption of vitamin _____ with aging.

    a. C
    b. D
    c. A
    d. E

18. Which of the following is provided by the *Senior Nutrition Program?*

    a. nutritious meals
    b. transportation
    c. assistance with housekeeping
    d. a and b
    e. b and c

19. Which of the following puts older adults at greatest risk of developing cataracts according to the latest scientific studies?

    a. excess food energy intake
    b. diets low in fruits and green vegetables
    c. excess intakes of milk and sugar
    d. deficiencies of riboflavin and zinc

Application Level Items:

20. Which of the following would the best snack choice for an active, normal weight child?

    a. flavored gelatin
    b. candy
    c. cola
    d. oatmeal cookies

21. Which of the following vegetables would be the most acceptable to a child?

    a. slightly overcooked green beans
    b. mixed vegetables
    c. broccoli
    d. bright green peas

22. Betsy is a two year old who has been on a food jag for five days. What is the best way to respond to Betsy's food jag?

    a. no response, since attention is a valuable reward
    b. serve tiny portions of many foods
    c. serve favored food items
    d. distract the child with friends at meals

23. To control dental caries, these foods should be used infrequently:

    a. cheese, apples, and hard rolls
    b. toast, chicken, and green beans
    c. chocolate milk, prunes, and candied sweet potatoes
    d. plain yogurt, eggs, and pizza

24. Which of the following snack foods would be most appropriate for a teenager trying to consume enough vitamin A?

    a. hard boiled eggs, bran muffin, and crackers
    b. carrot sticks, tomato juice, and dried apricots
    c. luncheon meat, whole-wheat bread, and celery sticks
    d. swiss cheese, crackers, and cantaloupe

25. Bessie is a 85 year old female who resides in a nursing home. She has a good appetite and consumes three cups of milk a day. However, Bessie is at risk for developing vitamin D deficiency because:

    a. she does not have adequate exposure to sunlight
    b. she does not consume an adequate amount of milk
    c. as she ages, her vitamin D synthesis declines
    d. a and b
    e. a and c

ANSWERS

SUMMING UP

(1) gender; (2) first; (3) 1000; (4) 300; (5) nutrients; (6) caffeine; (7) colas; (8) television; (9) adolescence; (10) fat; (11) snacks; (12) menstruation; (13) appetite; (14) behavior; (15) A; (16) calcium; (17) stress; (18) 80; (19) energy; (20) carbohydrate; (21) fats; (22) dehydration; (23) fiber; (24) A; (25) D; (26) vegetable; (27) zinc; (28) taste

CHAPTER GLOSSARY

Matching Exercise: (1) f; (2) j; (3) b; (4) l; (5) d; (6) o; (7) g; (8) q; (9) a; (10) m; (11) h; (12) k; (13) e; (14) n; (15) c; (16) i; (17) p; (18) s; (19) r

EXERCISES

Chapter Study Questions:

1. Television viewing requires no energy and seems to reduce the metabolic rate to levels below that of rest and it contributes to physical inactivity by consuming time that could be spent in more vigorous activities. Watching television also correlates with between-meal snacking and with eating the calorically dense and fatty foods most heavily advertised on children's programs. Finally, it encourages food behaviors that damage dental health.

2. Children who eat no breakfast perform poorly in tasks of concentration, their attention spans are shorter, they achieve lower test scores, and they are tardy or absent more often than their well-fed peers.

3. The individual should try to examine her total lifestyle, including diet, get adequate sleep, engage in physical activity, and try to moderate her intakes of caffeine, salt, alcohol, and any other abusable substances.

4. Foods low in fat are often rich in vitamins, minerals and phytochemicals and may help retard the development of cancer, atherosclerosis, obesity, and other diseases. A diet low in the fats of meats and dairy products may also improve some symptoms of arthritis.

5. The number of active cells in each organ decreases, which brings about a reduction in the body's metabolic rate. In addition, older people are not usually as physically active as younger people and their lean tissue diminishes.

Short Answer Questions:

1. (a) milk; (b) protein-rich foods; (c) vegetables; (d) fruits; (e) breads or other grains

2. (a) antibodies; (b) symptoms

3. (a) milk; (b) eggs; (c) peanuts; (d) tree nuts; (e) wheat; (f) soybeans; (g) fish; (h) shellfish

4. (a) desire for attention; (b) lack of sleep; (c) overstimulation; (d) too much television; (e) lack of exercise; (f) chronic hunger; (g) too much caffeine from colas or chocolate

5. (a) the metabolic rate; (b) glucose tolerance; (c) appetite; (d) food intake; (e) mood; (f) behavior

6. (a) iron; (b) calcium; (c) zinc; (d) vitamin D; (e) vitamin C

7. (a) iron; (b) zinc; (c) calcium

8. (a) many drink little or no vitamin D fortified milk; (b) many go day after day with no exposure to sunlight; (c) as people age, vitamin D synthesis declines

9. (a) abstinence from, or moderation in, alcohol use; (b) regular meals; (c) weight control; (d) adequate sleep; (e) abstinence from smoking; (f) regular physical activity

10. (a) loss of memory and reasoning power; (b) loss of ability to communicate; (c) loss of physical capabilities

Problem-Solving:

1. About 3 servings were consumed in the milk and milk product groups, which exceeds the two recommended servings. Two servings of meat foods were consumed, making this group adequate. The bread and cereal food group was not adequately represented, with a total of four servings versus the recommended six. Two servings of fruits were consumed, which was adequate, and only one vegetable was consumed, versus the three recommended. As a consequence, vitamins A and C, folate, carbohydrate, and fiber intake could be low for the day.

2.

	Low Caries Potential	High Caries Potential
a. plain yogurt	x	
b. sugared cereals		x
c. bagels	x	
d. dried fruit		x
e. popcorn	x	
f. glazed carrots		x
g. sugarless gum	x	
h. legumes	x	
i. fresh fruit	x	
j. chocolate milk		x

3.

	Higher	Lower	Same
a. energy		x	
b. fiber			x
c. vitamin A		x	
d. vitamin D	x		
e. protein			x

Controversy Questions:

1. The brain's cells cease communicating with each other

2. The protein and carbohydrate content of the meal

3. People are easily distracted from tests requiring vigilance and have slower reaction times; they also score lower on memory tests than at times of normal eating

4. Serotonin

5. Avoid foods extremely high in carbohydrates and low in protein in the hours before the test

SAMPLE TEST ITEMS

1. b (p. 478)	9. e (p. 489-490)	17. c (p. 493)
2. d (p. 482-483)	10. c (p. 488)	18. d (p. 499)
3. c (p. 480)	11. c (p. 492)	19. b (p. 494)
4. a (p. 484)	12. a (p. 490)	20. d (p. 475-476)
5. c (p. 486)	13. d (p. 493)	21. d (p. 476)
6. a (p. 489)	14. a (p. 491)	22. a (p. 477)
7. e (p. 476-477)	15. d (p. 492-495)	23. c (p. 484)
8. a (p. 478-479)	16. a (p. 498)	24. b (p. 489)
		25. e (p. 494)

CHAPTER 14

Food Safety and Food Technology

CHAPTER OBJECTIVES

After completing this chapter, you should be able to:

1. List and prioritize the five hazards in our food supply identified by the *Food and Drug Administration*.

2. Discuss how microbial food poisoning can be prevented and indicate which foods are particularly troublesome.

3. Describe the risks, if any, of the following in foods: natural toxins, environmental contaminants, pesticides, and hormone residues.

4. List five important food processing or preservation techniques and explain the effect they have on the nutrient content of foods.

5. Discuss the regulations concerning food additives and identify the special roles of the major classes of additives.

6. List the arguments for and against the use of organic foods and products of biotechnology. (Controversy 14)

KEY CONCEPTS

✓ Each year in the United States, many millions of people suffer from mild to life-threatening symptoms caused by food-borne illness.

✓ Industry employs sound practices to safeguard the commercial food supply from microbial threats. Still, incidents of commercial food-borne illness have caused widespread harm to health.

✓ To prevent food-borne illness, always remember that it can happen. Keep hot foods hot, keep cold foods cold, keep raw foods separate, and keep your hands and the kitchen clean.

✓ Some foods pose special microbial threats and so require special handling. Raw seafood is especially likely to be contaminated. Almost all types of food poisoning can be prevented by safe food preparation, storage, and cleanliness. Honey is unsafe for infants.

✓ Some special food safety concerns arise when traveling. To avoid food-borne illnesses, remember to boil it, cook it, peel it, or forget it.

✓ Natural foods contain natural toxins that can be hazardous if consumed in excess. To avoid poisoning by toxins, eat all foods in moderation, treat chemicals from all sources with respect, and choose a variety of foods.

✓ Persistent environmental contaminants pose a significant, but generally small, threat to the safety of food. An accidental spill can create an extreme hazard.

✓ Pesticides can be part of a safe food protection program, but can also be hazardous when handled or used inappropriately.

✓ The FDA tests for pesticide residues in both domestic and imported foods. Consumers can take steps to minimize their ingestion of pesticide residues in foods.

✓ Bovine somatotropin causes cattle to produce more meat and milk on less feed than untreated cattle. The FDA has deemed the practice safe, but consumer groups oppose it.

✓ Some nutrients are lost in food processing. Processing aims to protect food from microbial, oxidative, and enzymatic spoilage.

✓ Modified atmosphere packaging makes many fresh packaged foods available to consumers. MAP foods compare well to fresh foods in terms of nutrient quality. MAP foods may pose a threat of food-borne illness if not properly stored.

✓ Some water-soluble vitamins are destroyed by canning, but many more diffuse into the canning liquid. Fat-soluble vitamins and minerals are not affected by canning, but minerals also leach into canning liquid.

✓ Foods frozen promptly and kept frozen lose few nutrients.

✓ Commercially dried foods retain most of their nutrients, but home-dried foods often sustain dramatic losses.

✓ Extrusion involves heat and destroys nutrients.

✓ The FDA regulates the use of intentional additives. Additives must be safe, effective, and measurable in the final product. Additives on the GRAS list are assumed to be safe because they have long been used. Additives used must have wide margins of safety.

✓ Microbial food spoilage can be prevented by antimicrobial additives. Of these, sugar and salt have a long history of use. Nitrites added to meats have been associated with cancer in laboratory animals.

✓ Antioxidants prevent oxidative changes in foods that would lead to unacceptable discoloration and texture changes in the food. Ingestion of the antioxidant sulfites can cause problems for some people; BHT may offer antioxidant effects in the body.

✓ The addition of artificial colors is tightly controlled. Some people react adversely to the colorant tartrazine.

✓ Among flavorings added to foods, the flavor enhancer MSG has been determined to cause reactions in people with sensitivities to it.

✓ Incidental additives are substances that get into food during processing. They are well regulated, and most present no hazard.

✓ Nutrients are added to foods to enrich or to fortify them. These additives do not necessarily make the foods nutritious; they are rich only in the vitamins and minerals that have been added.

SUMMING UP

The (1) _____ is the major agency charged with monitoring the food supply.

According to the FDA, the food hazard which has the potential to cause the greatest harm to

people is (2) _____ food-borne illness.

The term *food-borne illness* refers either to food-borne infection or to food

(3) _____. The symptoms of one neurotoxin stand out as severe and commonly

fatal - those of (4) _____. The botulinum toxin is destroyed by (5) _____

so canned foods that have been boiled for ten minutes are generally safe from this threat.

Food can provide ideal conditions for (6) _____ to thrive or to produce

toxins. Disease-causing bacteria require warmth, (7) _____, and nutrients. To

defeat them, people who prepare food should keep hot food hot, keep cold food cold, keep raw

foods separate, and keep your hands and the (8) _____ clean. Foods that are high in

moisture and nutrients and those that are chopped or (9) _____ are especially favorable hosts for microbial growth. You cannot rely on your senses of smell and sight alone to warn you of hazards because most contamination is not detectable by (10) _____, taste, or appearance. Raw, unpasteurized (11) _____ and raw (12)_____ are especially likely to be contaminated.

A food (13) _____ is any substance occurring in food by accident, and the potential harmfulness depends in part on the extent to which it lingers in the environment or in the human body. To avoid toxicities from natural food constituents, such as solanine in potatoes, you should practice moderation, treat chemicals from all sources with respect, and choose a (14) _____ of foods. Risks to health from pesticide exposure are probably small for healthy adults, but (15) _____ may be more at risk for pesticide poisoning.

Canning, (16) _____, drying, extrusion and modified atmosphere processing are important techniques of processing foods. In general, frozen foods' nutrient contents are similar to those of (17) _____ foods and losses are minimal, although (18) _____ destroys some water-soluble vitamins.

Manufacturers use food (19) _____ to give foods desirable characteristics, including color, flavor, (20) _____, stability, enhanced nutrient composition, or resistance to spoilage. The use of additives is regulated by the FDA and additives must be safe, (21) _____ and detected and measured in the final food product. Additives included on the (22) _____ list are assumed to be safe because they have been long used.

Preservatives known as (23) _____ agents are used to protect foods from growth of microbes. The two best known and most widely used agents include sugar and (24)_____; both work by withdrawing (25) _____ from the food. Another group of antimicrobial agents, the (26) _____, are added to foods to preserve their color, to enhance their flavor, and to protect against bacterial growth, especially the deadly (27) _____ bacterium.

        Some foods go bad by undergoing changes in color and flavor caused by exposure to

(28) _____ in the air. Preservatives known as (29) _____ protect

food from this type of spoilage. Vitamin E and vitamin (30) _____ are used to

prevent oxidation, as well as sulfites, BHA, and (31) _____.

        Another class of additives is nutrients added to improve or maintain the

(32) _____ value of foods. Included among these are the nutrients added to

(33) _____ grains to enrich them, the (34) _____ added to salt,

vitamins A and (35) _____ added to dairy products, and the nutrients added to

fortified breakfast cereals.

CHAPTER GLOSSARY

Matching Exercise 1:

_____ 1. incidental additives

_____ 2. canning

_____ 3. modified atmosphere packaging

_____ 4. high-temperature-short-time principle

_____ 5. contaminant

_____ 6. MSG symptom complex

_____ 7. freezing

_____ 8. extrusion

_____ 9. GRAS list

_____ 10. drying

_____ 11. pesticides

_____ 12. additives

_____ 13. margin of safety

_____ 14. toxicity

_____ 15. ultrahigh temperature

_____ 16. organic foods

_____ 17. cross-contamination

a. the acute, temporary, and self-limiting reactions experienced by many people upon ingesting a large dose of MSG

b. preservation by removing sufficient water from food to inhibit microbial growth

c. substances that are added to foods, but are not normally consumed by themselves as foods

d. the ability of a substance to harm living organisms

e. preservation of a perishable food by packaging it in a gas-impermeable container from which air has been removed, or to which another gas mixture has been added

f. a heat process by which the form of food is changed, such as changing corn to corn chips; not a preservation measure

g. in reference to food additives, a zone between the concentration normally used and that at which a hazard exists

h. every 10°C (18°F) rise in processing temperature brings about an approximately tenfold increase in microbial destruction, while only doubling nutrient losses

i. substances that can get into food not through intentional introduction but as a result of contact with food during growing, processing, packaging, storing, or some other stage before the food is consumed

j. a list of food additives, established by the FDA, long in use and believed safe

k. short-time exposure of a food to temperatures above those normally used to sterilize it

l. preservation by lowering food temperature to the point at which life processes cease

m. chemicals used to control insects, diseases, weeds, fungi, and other pests on crops and around animals

n. preservation by killing all microorganisms present in food and sealing out air

o. any substance occurring in food by accident; not a normal food constituent

p. the contamination of a food through exposure to utensils, hands, or other surfaces that were previously in contact with a contaminated food.

q. products grown and processed without the use of synthetic chemicals such as pesticides, herbicides, fertilizers, and preservatives and without genetic engineering or irradiation

---

Matching Exercise 2:

_____ 1. neurotoxins

_____ 2. organic halogen

_____ 3. pasteurization

_____ 4. human somatotropin

_____ 5. biosensor

_____ 6. tolerance limit

_____ 7. growth hormone

_____ 8. botulism

_____ 9. biotechnology

_____ 10. hazard

_____ 11. bioaccumulation

_____ 12. heavy metal

_____ 13. Hazard Analysis Critical Control Point

_____ 14. bovine somatotropin

_____ 15. entertoxins

_____ 16. food-borne illness

_____ 17. foot-and-mouth disease

_____ 18. mad cow disease

a. the maximum amount of a residue permitted in a food when a pesticide is used according to label directions

b. any of a number of mineral ions such as mercury and lead

c. an organic compound containing one or more atoms of halogen - fluorine, chlorine, iodine, or bromine

d. a state of danger; used to refer to any circumstance in which harm is possible under normal conditions of use

e. poisons that act upon mucous membranes such as those of the digestive tract

f. a genetically altered microbe that provides a rapid, low-cost, and accurate test for toxic products of microbial agents in foods

g. the science that manipulates biological systems or organisms to modify their products or components or create new products

h. a systematic plan to identify and correct potential microbial hazards in the manufacturing, distribution, and commercial use of food products

i. the treatment of milk with heat sufficient to kill certain pathogens commonly transmitted through milk; not a sterilization process

j. a hormone (somatotropin) that promotes growth and that is produced naturally in the pituitary gland of the brain

k. poisons that act upon the cells of the nervous system

l. an often-fatal food poisoning caused by botulinum toxin, a toxin produced by bacteria that grow without oxygen in nonacidic canned foods

m. human growth hormone

n. the accumulation of a contaminant in the tissues of living things at higher and higher concentrations along the food chain

o. growth hormone of cattle which can be produced for agricultural use by genetic engineering

p. illness transmitted to human beings through food and water

q. an often-fatal illness of cattle affecting the nerves and brain; also called *bovine spongiform encephalopathy* (BSE)

r. a severely disabling contagious viral disease that threatens domestic and wild animals

EXERCISES

Answer these chapter study questions:

1. Why have food colors been more heavily criticized than almost any other group of additives?

2. Identify the steps which the FDA has taken to protect people who are allergic to sulfites.

3. Why are some foods more encouraging of microbial growth than others?

4. Explain what is meant by the statement that food processing involves a trade-off.

5. Why are vitamin C losses especially likely during the freezing process.

Complete these short answer questions:

1. Manufacturers use food additives to give foods desirable characteristics related to:

   a.
   b.
   c.
   d.
   e.
   f.

2. The best known and most widely used antimicrobial agents are:

   a.
   b.

3. Nitrites are added to foods to:

   a.
   b.
   c.

4. Four food products which commonly contain nutrient additives are:

   a.
   b.
   c.
   d.

5. Incidental food additives are substances that find their way into food as the result of some phase of:

   a.
   b.
   c.
   d.

6. Warning signs of botulism include:

   a.
   b.
   c.
   d.

7. Food preservation or processing techniques include:

   a.
   b.
   c.
   d.
   e.

8. The canning process is based on:

   a.
   b.

9. Advantages of drying as a food processing method include:

   a.
   b.
   c.

10. Four things which should be done in the kitchen in order to prevent food poisoning include:

    a.
    b.
    c.
    d.

Solve these problems:

For questions 1-5, match the types of food additives on the left with examples of the additives on the right.

_____ 1. antimicrobial agent   a. MSG

_____ 2. antioxidant   b. sulfites

_____ 3. artificial color   c. iodine

_____ 4. artificial flavor   d. nitrites

_____ 5. nutrient additive   e. tartrazine

Food Safety and Food Technology

For questions 6-9, for each food listed on the left, identify proper storage and/or cooking techniques to preserve the nutrient content, listed on the right.

_____ 6. milk

_____ 7. apples

_____ 8. cut orange

_____ 9. potatoes

a. chill immediately after picking and keep cold until used

b. cut after washing; add to water that is vigorously boiling

c. cover with airtight wrapper and store in refrigerator

d. store in cardboard or opaque plastic containers to protect riboflavin

Solve these controversy questions:

1. Which specific technologies cannot be used in the production of organic foods?

2. Would a consumer be able to detect a genetically modified food product in the grocery store? Why or why not?

3. What are plant pesticides and what are their limitations?

4. Are organic foods nutritionally superior to traditional foods? If so, in what way?

5. What are some of the potential health risks associated with organic foods?

STUDY AIDS

Use the following tables in your textbook as study aids: Table 14-5 on page 520; Table 14-8 on page 531; Table 14-9 on page 534; Table 14-10 on page 538.

SAMPLE TEST ITEMS

Comprehension Level Items:

1. Which of the following appears as the number one priority on the *Food and Drug Administration's* list of food hazards?

    a. pesticide residues
    b. food-borne illness
    c. intentional food additives
    d. naturally occurring toxicants

2. Substances that find their way into food as a result of production, processing, storage, or packaging are called _____ additives.

    a. incidental
    b. contaminant
    c. intentional
    d. direct

3.   FDA's authority over additives hinges primarily on their:

   a.   appropriate uses
   b.   effectiveness
   c.   safety
   d.   a and b
   e.   b and c

4.   If FDA approves an additive's use, that means the manufacturer can:

   a.   use it only in amounts specified by the FDA
   b.   add it to only those foods delineated by the FDA
   c.   add it in any amount to any food
   d.   a and b
   e.   b and c

5.   Which of the following is(are) true concerning the food color tartrazine?

   a.   it causes an allergic reaction in susceptible people
   b.   it must be mentioned on all labels of food that contain it
   c.   it appears in yellow-colored foods only
   d.   a and b
   e.   b and c

6.   MSG has been deemed safe for adults, but is kept out of foods for infants.

   a.   true
   b.   false

7.   Salt and sugar work as antimicrobial agents by:

   a.   removing oxygen from foods
   b.   withdrawing nutrients used as food by bacteria
   c.   withdrawing water from food
   d.   b and c
   e.   a and b

8.   Preservatives known as _____ protect food from undergoing changes by exposure to air.

   a.   glutamates
   b.   tartrazines
   c.   antimicrobials
   d.   antioxidants

9.   To reduce pesticide residues in foods you would:

   a.   trim the fat from meat
   b.   consume waxed vegetables without removing the wax
   c.   wash fresh produce in water
   d.   a and b
   e.   a and c

10. No food additives are permanently approved by the FDA.

    a. true
    b. false

11. To prevent bacterial growth, you should refrigerate foods immediately after serving a meal and definitely before _____ has(have) passed.

    a. 30 minutes
    b. 1 hour
    c. 2 hours
    d. 3 hours

12. Which of the following would be the safest food to pack for a picnic?

    a. carrot sticks
    b. pasta salad
    c. chicken salad
    d. Swiss cheese

13. A processing technique that preserves food by lowering food temperature to the point at which life processes cease is called:

    a. canning
    b. freezing
    c. drying
    d. extrusion

14. Which of the following is a special enemy of riboflavin?

    a. heat
    b. the canning process
    c. light
    d. ascorbic acid oxidase

15. You can use your senses of smell and sight alone to warn you of hazards and food contamination.

    a. true
    b. false

16. A mineral added when foods are canned is:

    a. potassium
    b. iron
    c. calcium
    d. sodium

17. Sulfites are highly destructive of:

    a. vitamin C
    b. riboflavin
    c. iron
    d. thiamin

18. Wooden cutting boards do not support microbial growth and therefore require no treatment.

    a. true
    b. false

19. To prevent traveler's diarrhea you would:

    a. wash hands before eating
    b. drink only bottled beverages
    c. wash fresh fruits under running water
    d. a and b
    e. b and c

Application Level Items:

20. Which of the following food products would be acceptable to purchase from the grocery store?

    a. a jar of jelly with a broken seal
    b. a solidly frozen package of spinach
    c. a can of tomatoes that is bulging
    d. a torn package of frozen green peas

21. Which of the following foods would be most susceptible to bacterial contamination?

    a. pork chop
    b. chicken breast
    c. meatloaf
    d. veal cutlet

22. Which of the following foods would be most appropriate to carry on a picnic?

    a. pimento cheese spread
    b. meatballs
    c. egg salad
    d. canned cheese spread

23. To prevent food poisoning you would:

    a. transfer leftovers to deep containers before refrigerating
    b. refrigerate perishables immediately when you get home
    c. thaw poultry in the refrigerator
    d. a and b
    e. b and c

24. The FDA approved the use of Aspartame as a sweetener several years ago. This means that:

    a. it can be added to only certain approved food products
    b. it can be added in unlimited quantities to foods
    c. it can be used forever in food products
    d. it can be placed on the GRAS list

25. You are interested in using a preservative which will protect a food from microbes and prevent the food from becoming hazardous to health. Which of the following would you use?

    a. ascorbate
    b. sulfites
    c. tartrazine
    d. nitrites

ANSWERS

SUMMING UP

(1) Food and Drug Administration; (2) microbial; (3) intoxication; (4) botulism; (5) heat; (6) bacteria; (7) moisture; (8) kitchen; (9) ground; (10) odor; (11) eggs, (12) seafood; (13) contaminant; (14) variety; (15) children; (16) freezing; (17) fresh; (18) canning; (19) additives; (20) texture; (21) effective; (22) GRAS; (23) antimicrobial; (24) salt; (25) water; (26) nitrites; (27) botulinum; (28) oxygen; (29) antioxidants; (30) C; (31) BHT; (32) nutritional; (33) refined; (34) iodine; (35) D

CHAPTER GLOSSARY

Matching Exercise 1: (1) i; (2) n; (3) e; (4) h; (5) o; (6) a; (7) l; (8) f; (9) j; (10) b; (11) m; (12) c; (13) g; (14) d; (15) k; (16) q; (17) p
Matching Exercise 2: (1) k; (2) c; (3) i; (4) m; (5) f; (6) a; (7) j; (8) l; (9) g; (10) d; (11) n; (12) b; (13) h; (14) o; (15) e; (16) p; (17) r; (18) q

EXERCISES

Chapter Study Questions:

1. Because they are dispensable and are used to make foods look pretty. In contrast, other food additives, such as preservatives, make foods safe.

2. It prohibits sulfite use on food intended to be consumed by infants; it requires that sulfite-containing foods and drugs list the additives on their labels to warn that sulfites are present.

3. Because the ideal conditions for bacteria to thrive include warmth, moisture, and nutrients; foods that are high in moisture and nutrients and those that are chopped or ground are especially favorable hosts for microbial growth.

4. Food processing makes food safer, gives it a longer usable lifetime than fresh food, or cuts preparation time; however, the cost is the loss of some vitamins and minerals.

5. Vitamin C losses occur whenever tissues are broken and exposed to the oxygen in the air. In the freezing process, vitamin C losses are likely to occur during the steps taken in preparation for freezing, including blanching, washing, trimming, or grinding.

Short Answer Questions:

1. (a) color; (b) flavor; (c) texture; (d) stability; (e) resistance to spoilage; (f) enhanced nutrient composition

2. (a) sugar; (b) salt

3. (a) preserve their color; (b) enhance their flavor by inhibiting rancidity; (c) protect against bacterial growth

4. (a) grains; (b) salt; (c) dairy products; (d) breakfast cereals

5. (a) production; (b) processing; (c) storage; (d) packaging

6. (a) double vision; (b) weak muscles; (c) difficulty swallowing; (d) difficulty breathing

7. (a) canning; (b) freezing; (c) drying; (d) extrusion; (e) modified atmosphere packaging

8. (a) time; (b) temperature

9. (a) it eliminates microbial spoilage; (b) it reduces the weight and volume of foods; (c) it does not cause major nutrient losses

10. (a) keep hot foods hot; (b) keep cold foods cold; (c) keep your hands and the kitchen clean; (d) keep raw food separate

Problem-Solving:

(1) d; (2) b; (3) e; (4) a; (5) c; (6) d; (7) a; (8) c; (9) b

Controversy Questions:

1. Irradiation and biotechnology

2. No, because no label is required for genetically modified products

3. Plant pesticides are a group of pesticides made by the plants themselves; limitations include a lack of control of pests not killed by the plant pesticide, the high cost of producing the transgenic plants, and the development of resistance to the pesticide among the target population of insects.

4. Some findings suggest that organic foods have slightly greater vitamin C content, lower nitrate, and somewhat improved protein quality but the differences were small and not significant to human health.

5. The use of improperly composted animal manure fertilizer may expose consumers to E. coli; unpasteurized organic juices, milk and cheese may also constitute microbial hazards because pasteurization is required to kill disease-causing microorganisms in these foods; also organic foods contain no preservatives and tend to spoil faster than other foods

SAMPLE TEST ITEMS

1. b (p. 510)	9. e (p. 534)	17. d (p. 541)
2. a (p. 542)	10. a (p. 539)	18. b (p. 518)
3. e (p. 539)	11. c (p. 518)	19. d (p. 523-524)
4. d (p. 539)	12. a (p. 523)	20. b (p. 516)
5. d (p. 542)	13. b (p. 537)	21. c (p. 520)
6. a (p. 542)	14. c (p. 536)	22. d (p. 523)
7. c (p. 540)	15. b (p. 518)	23. e (p. 518)
8. d (p. 541)	16. d (p. 537)	24. a (p. 539-540)
		25. d (p. 540)

CHAPTER 15

Hunger and the Global Environment

CHAPTER OBJECTIVES

After completing this chapter, you should be able to:

1. Discuss some of forces that threaten world food production and distribution in the next decade.

2. Distinguish between the following terms: hunger, food insecurity, food poverty, and food shortage.

3. List some of the U.S. government programs designed to relieve poverty and hunger and discuss their effectiveness.

4. Compare the causes of hunger in the United States and in developing countries and explain the roles played by food shortages, chronic hunger, and the diminishing world food supply.

5. Explain how relieving poverty and overpopulation will help alleviate environmental degradation and hunger.

6. List some of the environmentally conscious food shopping and cooking activities consumers can choose to minimize the impacts on the environment.

7. Discuss some of the environmental and social costs of agriculture and the food industry and indicate possible solutions that would enable both agribusiness and the environment to survive. (Controversy 15)

KEY CONCEPTS

✓ The world's chronically hungry people suffer the effects of undernutrition, and many in the United States live with food insecurity. Many forces combine to threaten the world's future food supply and its distribution.

✓ Chronic hunger causes many deaths worldwide, especially among children. Intermittent hunger is frequently seen in U.S. children. The immediate cause of hunger is poverty.

✓ Poverty and hunger coexist with affluence and bounty in the United States, not only among the unemployed, but also among working people. Government programs to relieve poverty and hunger are tremendously helpful, if not fully successful.

✓ Natural causes such as drought, flood, and pests and social causes such as armed conflicts and overpopulation all contribute to hunger and poverty in developing countries. To meet future demands for food, technology must continue to improve food production, food must be fairly distributed, and birth rates need to decline. The world's women and girls are major allies in the effort to fight hunger.

✓ Environmental degradation caused by the impacts of growing numbers of people is threatening the world's future ability to feed all of its citizens. Improvements in agriculture can no longer keep up with people's growing numbers. Human population growth is an urgent concern. Controlling population growth requires improving people's economic status and providing them with health care, education, and family planning.

✓ Government, business, educators, and all individuals have many opportunities to promote sustainability worldwide and wise resource use at home.

SUMMING UP

In the United States, over (1) _____ million children do not know where their next

meal is coming from or when it will come. (2) _____ is a condition of uncertain

access to food of sufficient quality or quantity. The primary cause of hunger in developed nations

is (3) _____. In the US food poverty affects not only the chronic poor but also the

so-called (4) _____ poor.

Hunger and poverty interact with a third force, which is (5)_____degradation.

One element of this degradation is (6) _____ which is affecting agriculture in every

nation. The only way to enable the world's output to keep pace with people's growing numbers is

(7) _____ control.

Population growth, (8) _____ and environmental degradation combine to

worsen each other. Breaking the cycle requires improving the (9) _____ status of the people and providing them with health care, (10) _____ , and family planning.

Both rich and poor nations play key roles in solving the world's environmental, poverty, and

(11) _____ problems. Poor nations need to make (12) _____ technology

and information more widely available, (13)_____ their citizens and adopt

(14) _____ development practices that slow the destruction of their forests,

waterways and soil. Rich nations need to stem their wasteful and polluting uses of resources and

(15) _____ , which are contributing to global environmental degradation.

Many nations now agree that improvement of all nation's (16) _____ is a

prerequisite to meeting the world's urgent needs. At a summit of over 100 nations, many agreed

to a set of principles of (17) _____ development. The conference defined

sustainable development as development that would meet both the economic and

(18) _____ needs of present and future generations.

Consumers can choose to minimize negative impacts on the (19) _____ in

many ways. Small decisions each day, such as making fewer (20) _____ trips,

choosing foods low on the (21) _____, and buying locally grown foods, can add up

to large impacts on the environment. In addition, consumers can buy bulk items with minimal

(22)_____ , use (23) _____ cooking methods, and purchase the

most efficient large (24) _____ possible. Products bearing the US government's

(25) _____logo rank highest for energy efficiency.

CHAPTER GLOSSARY

Matching Exercise:

_____ 1. food poverty

_____ 2. famine

_____ 3. food insecurity

_____ 4. world food supply

_____ 5. gleaning

_____ 6. hunger

_____ 7. sustainable

_____ 8. oral rehydration therapy

_____ 9. carrying capacity

_____ 10. food shortage

a. lack or shortage of basic foods needed to provide the energy and nutrients that support health

b. oral fluid replacement for children with severe diarrhea caused by infectious disease

c. widespread, scarcity of food in an area that causes starvation and death in a large portion of the population

d. the recovery of excess food from various sources including restaurants, hotels, farms and supermarkets

e. hunger occurring when an area of the world lacks enough total food to feed its people

f. the quantity of food, including stores from previous harvests, available to the world's people at a given time

g. able to continue indefinitely; the term refers to the use of resources at such a rate that the earth can keep on replacing them

h. hunger occurring when enough food exists in an area but some of the people cannot obtain it because they lack money, they are being deprived for political reasons, they live in a country at war, or because of other problems such as lack of transportation

i. the total number of living organisms that a given environment can support without deteriorating in quality

j. the condition of uncertain access to food of sufficient quality or quantity

EXERCISES

Answer these chapter study questions:

1. What is meant by the term *sustainable* and what is an example?

2. Why is it environmentally beneficial to eat low on the food chain?

3. Why are fast cooking methods recommended as one step consumers should take to minimize negative impacts on the environment? What are some examples?

4. Describe what is meant by the statement that hunger, poverty, and environmental degradation all interact with each other.

5. Why do people living in poverty bear more children?

Complete these short answer questions:

1. Some of the forces threatening world food production and distribution in the next decade include:

    a.   f.
    b.   g.
    c.   h.
    d.   i.
    e.   j.

2. The primary cause of hunger in developed nations is _____.

3. Natural causes of famine include:

    a.
    b.
    c.

4. Fast cooking methods that use less energy than conventional stovetop cooking methods include:

    a.
    b.
    c.

5. To minimize the energy a refrigerator uses you would:

    a.
    b.
    c.

6. To solve the world's environmental, poverty, and hunger problems, the poor nations need to:

    a.
    b.
    c.
    d.

7. The death rate falls when people attain better access to:

    a.
    b.
    c.

8. Food stamp coupons cannot be used to purchase:

    a.
    b.
    c.
    d.

9. To solve the world's environmental, poverty, and hunger problems, the rich nations need to_____.

10. In the US, the chronic poor include::

   a.
   b.
   c.
   d.

Solve these problems:

Place an x next to each of the behaviors below which are environmentally conscious.

_____ car pool to the grocery store
_____ eat high on the food chain
_____ buy foods which are locally grown
_____ buy canned beef products
_____ select fish such as tuna, swordfish, and shark
_____ buy items in bulk
_____ use plastic bags instead of paper ones
_____ use the microwave for cooking

Solve these controversy questions:

1. What is agribusiness?

2. How does massive fossil fuel use threaten our planet?

3. What is the problem with raising animals in concentrated areas such as cattle feed lots?

4. What is meant by *integrated pest management?*

5. How can biotechnology lead to economic, environmental, and agricultural benefits?

SAMPLE TEST ITEMS

Comprehension Level Items:

1. Which of the following trends are expected to continue into the next decade??

    a. more children are being born than are dying of malnutrition
    b. global warming is decreasing
    c. the ozone layer is growing thicker
    d. the number of forests is increasing

2. Which of the following is(are) example(s) of the working poor in the US?

    a. the unskilled
    b. displaced farm families
    c. former blue collar workers forced out of their trades
    d. a and b
    e. b and c

3. The term *sustainable* means the ability to continue indefinitely.

    a. true
    b. false

4. Which of the following is a condition of uncertain access to food of sufficient quality or quantity?

    a. hunger
    b. food poverty
    c. food shortage
    d. food insecurity

5. Which of the following is the leading cause of blindness in the world's young children?

    a. vitamin A deficiency
    b. iodine deficiency
    c. vitamin C deficiency
    d. protein deficiency

6. If you are a meat eater, which of the following recommendations would you follow in order to be environmentally conscious?

    a. select canned corn beef
    b. choose chicken from local farms
    c. select small fish
    d. a and b
    e. b and c

7. Which of the following fish species is endangered by overfishing?

    a. snapper
    b. flounder
    c. salmon
    d. shark

8. Which of these types of bags is the best choice from an environmental perspective?

    a. paper
    b. plastic
    c. cloth
    d. a and b
    e. b and c

9. Locally grown foods require less transportation, packaging, and refrigeration.

    a. true
    b. false

10. Which of the following packaging techniques for processed foods is the most environmentally advantageous?

    a. meat wrapped in butcher paper
    b. eggs in foam cartons
    c. juices in small individual cartons
    d. grain products in separate little packages

11. Which of the following cooking aids is the best choice from an environmental perspective?

   a.   paper towels
   b.   plastic wrap
   c.   dishcloths
   d.   aluminum foil

12. Refrigerators are one of the kitchen appliances that use the most energy in most people's homes.

   a.   true
   b.   false

13. In the United States, hunger is the result of:

   a.   food insecurity
   b.   food shortage
   c.   famine
   d.   food poverty

14. In the United States, one of every _____ Americans receives food assistance of some kind.

   a.   2
   b.   4
   c.   6
   d.   10

15. Hunger is not always easy to recognize.

   a.   true
   b.   false

16. To help solve the world's environmental, poverty, and hunger problems, the poor nations should:

   a.   make contraceptive technology more widely available
   b.   educate their citizens
   c.   stem their wasteful uses of resources and energy
   d.   a and b
   e.   b and c

17. Example(s) of the chronic poor include(s):

   a.   migrant workers
   b.   the homeless
   c.   displaced farm families
   d.   a and b
   e.   b and c

18. Recipients can use food stamps to purchase:

    a. alcohol
    b. cleaning items
    c. seeds
    d. tobacco

19. Food recovery, or gleaning, from private industry has become a national priority.

    a. true
    b. false

20. Which of the following is a prerequisite to curbing population growth?

    a. relieving poverty
    b. inventing effective birth control measures
    c. alleviating hunger
    d. a and b
    e. a and c

Application Level Items:

21. Which of the following would you do to be an environmentally conscious food shopper?

    a. buy bulk items with minimal packaging
    b. choose chicken over beef
    c. eat canned chili
    d. choose fish which has been flown in from far away

22. By purchasing fresh foods grown locally you are:

    a. selecting nutritionally superior foods
    b. saving money
    c. helping the local economy
    d. minimizing negative impacts on the environment

23. You want to cook a whole roast for dinner. Which of the following would be the safest and best way to save energy?

    a. use the microwave
    b. use the oven
    c. use the outdoor gas grill
    d. use the pressure cooker

24. To solve the world's environmental, poverty, and hunger problems, rich nations must:

    a. gain control of their population growth
    b. stem their wasteful and polluting uses of resources and energy
    c. reverse the destruction of their environmental resources
    d. educate their citizens

25. Which of the following steps should be taken to relieve poverty and environmental degradation worldwide?

    a. ease the debt burden that many poor nations face
    b. adopt sustainable development practices that slow destruction of waterways, forests, and soil
    c. emphasize technology-intensive methods of harvesting the resources of developing countries
    d. a and b
    e. b and c

ANSWERS

SUMMING UP

(1) nine; (2) food insecurity; (3) food poverty; (4) working; (5) environmental;
(6) soil erosion; (7) population; (8) poverty; (9) economic; (10) education;
(11) hunger; (12) contraceptive; (13) educate; (14) sustainable; (15) energy;
(16) economies; (17) sustainable; (18) environmental; (19) environment; (20) shopping;
(21) food chain; (22) packaging; (23) fast; (24) appliances; (25) Energy Star

CHAPTER GLOSSARY

Matching Exercise: (1) h; (2) c; (3) j; (4) f; (5) d; (6) a; (7) g; (8) b; (9) i; (10) e

EXERCISES

Chapter Study Questions:

1. The term *sustainable* refers to the use of resources at such a rate that the earth can keep on replacing them. An example would be cutting trees no faster than new ones grow.

2. Because growing animals for their meat and dairy products by feeding them grain uses more land and other resources than growing grain and other crops for direct use by people. In addition, animals use more water, add more pollution to waterways, and, in general, cause destruction of more native vegetation and wildlife than equivalent amounts of plants.

3. Fast cooking methods use less energy than conventional stovetop or oven cooking methods. Examples include stir-frying, pressure cooking, and microwaving.

4. Poor people often destroy the resources they need for survival, such as soil and forests. When they cut the trees for firewood or timber to sell, they lose the soil to erosion and without these resources, they become poorer still. Thus, poverty causes environmental ruin and hunger grows from environmental ruin.

5. Poverty and hunger are correlated with lack of education which includes lack of knowledge on how to control family size. Also, families depend on children to farm the land, haul water, and care for adults in their old age. Many young children living in poverty also die from disease or other causes, in which case parents choose to have many children as a form of "insurance" that some will survive to adulthood.

Short Answer Questions:

1. (a) hunger, poverty, and population growth; (b) loss of food-producing land; (c) accelerating fossil fuel use; (d) increasing air pollution; (e) atmosphere and climate changes, droughts, and floods; (f) ozone loss from the outer atmosphere; (g) water shortages; (h) deforestation and desertification; (i) ocean pollution; (j) extinctions of species

2. food poverty

3. (a) drought; (b) flood; (c) pests

4. (a) stir-frying; (b) pressure cooking; (c) microwaving

5. (a) keep it set at 37-40° F; (b) clean the coils and the insulating gaskets around the door regularly; (c) keep it in good repair

6. (a) make contraceptive technology and information more widely available; (b) educate their citizens; (c) assist the poor; (d) adopt sustainable development practices that slow and reverse the destruction of their forests, waterways, and soil

7. (a) health care; (b) family planning; (c) education

8. (a) tobacco; (b) cleaning items; (c) alcohol; (d) nonfood items

9. stem their wasteful and polluting uses of resources and energy

10. (a) migrant workers; (b) the unskilled and unemployed; (c) the homeless; (d) some elderly

Problem-Solving:

X car pool to the grocery store
___ eat high on the food chain
X buy foods which are locally grown
___ buy canned beef products
___ select fish such as tuna, swordfish, and shark
X buy items in bulk
___ use plastic bags instead of paper ones
X use the microwave for cooking

Controversy Questions:

1. Agriculture that is practiced on a massive scale by large corporations owing vast acreages and employing intensive technologies, fuel and chemical inputs

2. By causing ozone depletion, water pollution, ocean pollution, and other ills and by making global warming likely

3. Large masses of animal waste are produced and they leach into local soils and water supplies, polluting them

4. Farmers using this system employ many techniques, such as crop rotation and natural predators, to control pests rather than relying on heavy use of pesticides alone

5. By shrinking the acreage needed for crops, reducing soil losses, minimizing use of chemical insecticides, and bettering crop protection

SAMPLE TEST ITEMS

1. a (p. 559-560)
2. e (p. 560)
3. a (p. 567)
4. d (p. 559)
5. a (p. 560)
6. e (p. 569)
7. d (p. 565)
8. c (p. 569)

9. a (p. 569)
10. a (p. 569)
11. c (p. 569)
12. a (p. 570)
13. d (p. 560)
14. c (p. 561)
15. a (p. 560)
16. d (p. 567)

17. d (p. 560)
18. c (p. 561)
19. a (p. 562)
20. e (p. 567)
21. a (p. 569)
22. d (p. 569)
23. d (p. 569)
24. b (p. 567)
25. b (p. 568)